LONG-TERM CARE
SKILLED
SERVICES

Applying Medicare's Rules to Clinical Practice

Elizabeth Malzahn

Elizabeth Malzahn, Author
Adrienne Trivers, Managing Editor
Jamie Carmichael, Associate Group Publisher
Emily Sheahan, Group Publisher
Mike Mirabello, Senior Graphic Artist
Matt Sharpe, Production Supervisor
Shane Katz, Art Director
Jean St. Pierre, Senior Director of Operations

Advice given is general. Readers should consult professional counsel for specific legal, ethical, or clinical questions.

Arrangements can be made for quantity discounts. For more information, contact:

HCPro, Inc.
75 Sylvan Street, Suite A-101
Danvers, MA 01923
Telephone: 800/650-6787 or 781/639-1872
Fax: 800/639-8511
E-mail: *customerservice@hcpro.com*

Visit HCPro online at:
www.hcpro.com and www.hcmarketplace.com

Contents

Contents

Elizabeth Malzahn

Elizabeth Malzahn, national director of healthcare for Covenant Retirement Communities, has extensive experience in skilled nursing operations, including third-party billing, revenue enhancement, and regulatory compliance.

After graduating from Culver-Stockton College with a bachelor's degree in accounting, Malzahn spent more than 14 years working in nursing home operations where she specialized in Medicare billing. She then moved to a Chicago-based public accounting and consulting firm where she spent 10 years specializing in healthcare.

As the skilled nursing and assisted living subject-matter expert for Covenant Retirement Communities, Malzahn oversees the skilled nursing and assisted living operations at the senior services provider's 13 campuses nationwide.

An authority on healthcare regulation and compliance, Malzahn conducts training programs for Covenant Retirement Communities as well as for HCPro, and for national and state nonprofit healthcare organizations.

Foreword

Industry Scope

As the skilled nursing industry transforms to meet the changing needs of beneficiaries, we are seeing an increase in utilization of SNF Medicare days. The number of SNF providers has remained relatively stable from 2001 to 2009, but total Medicare expenditures increased during that period from $12.1 billion to over $25 billion. Even more striking in 2009, the average number of days per admission was reduced to 35 days and the average reimbursement for those days still hovers at $12,600 or, in simpler terms, about $358 per day.

Reimbursement drives healthcare today and forces Medicare to ensure that SNFs adhere to the multitude of rules and regulations to prevent unnecessary expenditures in entitlement plans. Scrutiny by multiple regulators is increasing along with the growing expenditure of dollars. Medicare in a SNF can be broken down into three distinct components: eligibility, coverage, and payment. This book deals with the ins and outs of skilled coverage.

Frequent Obstacles Encountered

Too often, we hear, "Mrs. A's therapy is done, so we're going to cut her from skilled service." We get caught up in the notion that in order to be skilled, a resident must be receiving therapy or intensive nursing care. Failure to recognize other skills or skilled services prompts discontinuing or "cutting" the patient from skilled care too soon, depriving him or her of his or her skilled benefit and depriving the facility of needed revenue.

Sometimes, only because the patient classifies into a payment or resource utilization group (RUG) category, skilled coverage is continued, even though there is not a daily skilled need! Although the two aspects—coverage and payment—are related and interdependent, a patient must still meet all the skilled coverage guidelines as well as classify into a RUG category in order to receive a benefit. Sometimes, the CMS Common Working File has not been properly notified or updated. Therefore, it will not calculate the required 60-day break in skilled service that is necessary to generate a new benefit period. It could be the result of not submitting the correct claim information from your billing department or the billing department of another institution.

Experiment in your own facility. Determine the actual criteria and process staff use in your facility to determine who is "skilled" and who is not. Ask staff members on various shifts which patients under their care are "skilled" and why. Ask them to identify the daily skilled needs. Now check the documentation. Does the documentation truly support "skilled need and skilled care"? Does it support the benefit period? Does the patient also classify for a RUG payment category? If responses vary among staff, as I suspect they will, documentation of those patients will probably not be accurate or complete and will not withstand scrutiny from medical review.

It all needs to work together: coverage, payment, and supporting documentation

Frequently, staff wants a magic list or check-off sheet of what defines a skilled resident. Unfortunately, because the combinations of treatments, needs, diagnosis, care, and physician's orders are infinite, no such list exists. So let's try to simplify the process, while adhering to the Medicare rules. Facility practice may innocently deviate from the regulations, placing Medicare dollars at risk, and limiting optimal revenue.

The goal in this volume is to return to basics. Review the rules and regulations for skilled coverage and learn to apply them consistently, adjusting facility practices as necessary. This will ensure coverage for those that meet the requirements, allow the facility to manage the daily operations that affect skilled coverage, and direct necessary documentation.

The information presented in this manual is not hard to follow. With a complete understanding of how to handle the major pain points associated with skilled services—which this book will provide—a SNF will put itself in the best possible position to receive proper Medicare reimbursement. We hope you find this text useful in navigating the tedious world of Medicare coverage in a SNF.

—*Diane Brown, Regulatory Specialist*
HCPro, Inc.

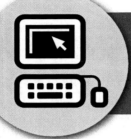

DOWNLOAD YOUR MATERIALS NOW

You can download your materials at the following URL:

www.hcpro.com/downloads/9310

Thank you for purchasing this product!

HCPro

CHAPTER

1

Breaking Down the Regulations

Rules and Regulations

The Social Security Act (42. USC, Chapter 7)

Once a law is passed, it is codified in the United States Code (USC) and published on the Government Printing Office website (GPO Access). The original Social Security Act was signed on August 14, 1935, by Franklin D. Roosevelt's administration as part of the New Deal. This act was the first legislation that identified the need for protection of the elderly in our country and was funded through an employee and employer contribution to a new payroll tax called Federal Insurance Contributions Act (FICA). The act was amended in 1965 to include the Medicare program. Since 1965, Congress has enacted many new provisions, considered to be amendments to the act. The subchapters identified as follows outline the areas and the individuals impacted by the original act and subsequent amendments:

- Subchapter I—Grants to states for old-age assistance

- Subchapter II—Federal old-age, survivors, and disability insurance benefits

- Subchapter III—Grants to states for unemployment compensation administration

- Subchapter IV—Grants to states for aid and services to needy families with children and for child-welfare services

- Subchapter V—Maternal and child health services block grant

- Subchapter VI—Temporary state fiscal relief

- Subchapter VII—Administration

Long-Term Care Skilled Services   © 2011 HCPro, Inc.   **1**

- Subchapter VIII—Special benefits for certain World War II veterans

- Subchapter IX—Employment security administrative financing

- Subchapter X—Grants to states for aid to the blind

- Subchapter XI—General provisions, peer review, and administrative simplification

- Subchapter XII—Advances to state unemployment funds

- Subchapter XIII—Reconversion unemployment benefits for seamen

- Subchapter XIV—Grants to states for aid to permanently and totally disabled

- Subchapter XV—Unemployment compensation for federal employees

- Subchapter XVI—Supplemental security income for aged, blind, and disabled

- Subchapter XVII—Grants for planning comprehensive action to combat mental retardation

- Subchapter XVIII—Health insurance for aged and disabled

- Subchapter XIX—Grants to states for medical assistance programs

- Subchapter XX—Block grants to states for social services

- Subchapter XXI—State Children's Health Insurance Program (SCHIP)

As previously identified, the Medicare program regulations reside in Subchapter XVII and the Medicaid program regulations reside in Subchapter XIX. This is where the terms Title 18 and Title 19 referring to Medicare and Medicaid, respectfully, is derived.

Amendments to the act

Such amendments and laws include the following:

- Social Security Amendments of 1965: These amendments, signed into law in 1965 by President Lyndon B. Johnson, created both the Medicare and Medicaid programs.

- The Omnibus Reconciliation Act (1987): This was the most significant legislation passed by President Ronald Reagan since the Medicare and Medicaid programs were created in 1965. This act demanded that nursing homes provide an environment that allows its residents to "attain and maintain their highest practicable physical, mental and psychosocial well-being" (Omnibus Reconciliation Act).

- Balanced Budget Act (BBA; 1997): This act was introduced to assist in balancing the Medicare budget by 2002. There were significant payment revisions to skilled nursing facilities (SNF). This act also included the introduction of the prospective payment system (PPS) and consolidated billing. In addition to making modifications for the current reimbursement under traditional Medicare, this act also introduced the Medicare+Choice Program options, as well as additional preventative care benefits for Medicare beneficiaries.

- Medicare, Medicaid, and SCHIP Balanced Budget Refinement Act (1999): This act was a revision to the BBA from 1997 that impacted SNFs as follows:

  - Increase in payment for higher cost residents

  - Increase to federal rates for all residents

  - Increase to the facility-specific rates for all SNFs

- Medicare, Medicaid, and SCHIP Benefits Improvement and Protection Act (2000): This act included additional reimbursement modifications related to the market-basket reduction previously made, removed some ineffective legislation related to consolidated billing requirements for non-Part A stays, and made some additional revisions to the Medicare+Choice Program requirements. There were also several other areas with an impact to skilled services in a long-term care setting:

  - Waived the 24-month waiting period for individuals with amyotrophic lateral sclerosis to qualify for Medicare benefits

  - Provided additional clarification and coverage for certain drugs and biologicals

  - Substantially revised the Medicare appeals process for both providers and beneficiaries and introduced the qualified independent contractors (QIC) who were contracted for an initial three-year agreement to conduct appeal reconsideration requests

- Medicare Prescription Drug, Improvement and Modernization Act (2003): This act provided what is commonly referred to in the industry as the "largest overhaul of Medicare in the program's 38-year history." The following are the highlights of this act impacting SNFs:

  - Introduction of a prescription drug benefit and entitlement to Medicare beneficiaries, commonly called Medicare Part D

  - Significant legislation impacting the Medicare+Choice Program, which also changed the name of this program to Medicare Advantage

  - A complete restructuring in the way that Medicare Part A and Part B claims are processed with the gradual replacement of fiscal intermediaries (FI) and carriers with Medicare Administrative Contractors (MAC)

Regulations Developed by CMS

Medicare regulation (e.g., 42 CFR § 409.33)

Once passed, such laws are then codified into regulation by the Centers for Medicare & Medicaid Services (CMS). The *Code of Federal Regulations (CFR)* is accessible on the Government Printing Office website. All regulations must be published initially in the Federal Register before enactment, and any changes to regulations must also be published in the Federal Register. Modifications and updates to the payment portion of the *CFR* are made at least once each year.

CMS manuals

Once the federal rules and regulations are in place, the information flows down to the intermediaries and providers. Effective October 1, 2003, CMS replaced its "paper-based" manual system with a new "Internet-only manual" (IOM) system. According to the Introduction (Pub. 100), "The process includes the streamlining, updating, and consolidating of CMS' various program instructions into an electronic Web-based manual system for all users. The new system is called the online CMS manual system and is located at *www.cms.hhs.gov/manuals*."

The CMS resource previously listed also includes the link to the Future Updates for the IOM to allow users to have the most up-to-date and current information related to the IOMs.

The following IOMs should be of particular relevance for questions relating to Medicare coverage, coding, billing, and payment for physician services:

- Pub. 100-01: *Medicare General Information, Eligibility, and Entitlement*

- Pub. 100-02: *Medicare Benefit Policy Manual* (basic coverage rules)

- Pub. 100-03: *Medicare National Coverage Determinations Manual* (national coverage decisions)

- Pub. 100-04: *Medicare Claims Processing Manual*

- Pub. 100-05: *Medicare Secondary Payer Manual*

- Pub. 100-16: *Medicare Managed Care Manual*

CMS program transmittals

CMS constantly issues new interpretations, mandates, and rules through program transmittals, which can create anxiety for someone who is trying to understand the world of skilled nursing. A transmittal may, for instance, clarify a rule related to Medicare, such as consolidated billing or how to bill for a particular item. According to CMS' definition:

> *Program transmittals are used to communicate new or changed policies, and/or procedures that are being incorporated into a specific Centers for Medicare & Medicaid services (CMS) program manual. The cover page (or transmittal page) summarizes the new changed material, specifying what is changed.*

In general, there are three types of transmittals:

- Transmittals announcing changes to the substantive manuals: These typically include a "red-lined" copy of revised manual sections.

- One-time notification (OTN) transmittals: These communicate information but do not change the manuals.

  - Some OTN transmittals are "tied" to particular manuals and include the manual name in the transmittal number.

  - Other OTN transmittals are more global in nature and are not tied to any particular substantive manual. Rather, they are tied to the *OTN Manual* (Pub. 100-20), which is really more of a filing system than a substantive manual. These transmittals include "OTN" in the transmittal number.

- Recurring update notification transmittals: These communicate information that changes on a regular schedule (e.g., code lists, edit specifications), but, like OTN transmittals, they do not make changes to the substantive manuals. They are typically tied to a particular substantive manual and are also tied to the *Recurring Update Notification Manual* (Pub. 100-21), which is more of a filing system than a true manual.

Medicare Learning Network articles

In addition to the manuals and transmittals, CMS publishes a series of articles called Medicare Learning Network (MLN) articles. These articles are intended to provide practical operational information about the Medicare program. Many of the articles are designed to accompany and/or explain recent CMS transmittals. CMS describes the articles as follows:

> The Centers for Medicare & Medicaid Services (CMS) is committed to partnering with the Medicare physician, provider, and supplier communities to ensure that Medicare beneficiaries receive all of the healthcare services to which they are entitled. CMS assists the healthcare community in providing the best services to Medicare beneficiaries by ensuring that healthcare professionals have ready access to Medicare coverage and reimbursement rules in a brief, accurate, and easy-to-understand format. To help meet this goal, CMS has developed MLN Matters.

The articles are grouped by year and each year has an index available to make searching for specific topics easier.

Coverage Determinations

Coverage of items or services under the Medicare benefit is limited to items that are reasonable and necessary and for the treatment of an illness or injury in the most appropriate care setting. Coverage decisions fall into two main categories:

- National coverage determination (NCD)

- Local coverage determination (LCD)

NCDs

By CMS' definition, NCDs "are made through an evidence-based process, with opportunities for public participation. In some cases, CMS' own research is supplemented by an outside technology assessment and/or consultation with the Medicare Evidence Development & Coverage Advisory Committee (MEDCAC)."

The problem, however, is that not all FIs, carriers, or MACs act completely alike. Each can interpret CMS' transmittals, CMS' mandates, and the federal government's laws differently than the others do.

As a result, the government has to provide the "final word" when a definitive clarification of a coverage situation is missing. These clarifications are accomplished through the National Coverage Decision Committee, which issues NCDs.

FIGURE

1.1

Medicare national coverage process

The Medicare National Coverage Process is a nine (9) month process. For the initial six (6) months, the following phases often include the following in the order listed:

| Preliminary Discussions | Benefit Category | National Coverage Request | Staff Review | External Technology Assessment And / Or Medicare Coverage Advisory Committee |

| Staff Review | Draft Decision Memorandum Posted |

The final three (3) months of the Medicare National Coverage Process include a thirty (30) day Public Comments phase, followed by a sixty (60) day requirement to complete the Final Decision Memorandum and Implementation Instructions phase.

| Public Comments | Final Decision Memorandum and Implementation Instructions |

Upon completion of the Final Decision Memorandum and Implementation Instructions phase, two (2) further phases are possible: the Final Decision Memorandum and Implementation phase initiates an appeal or the Reconsideration phase will further initiate the Preliminary Discussions phase.

| Final Decision Memorandum and Implementation Instructions | Department Appeals Board |

Or

| Final Decision Memorandum and Implementation Instructions | Reconsideration | Preliminary Discussions |

  Long-Term Care Skilled Services

LCDs

To complicate matters further, each FI, carrier, or MAC typically interprets the rules and then issues its policy based on that interpretation. Each organization's policy offers a vast array of interpretations of specific rules and regulations and can serve as a great educational tool.

According to Section 1869(f)(2)(B) of the Social Security Act, "For purposes of this section, the term 'local coverage determination' means a determination by a fiscal intermediary or carrier under part A or part B, as applicable, respecting whether or not a particular item or service is covered on an intermediary- or carrier-wide basis under such parts." LCDs contain conditions of coverage as reasonable and necessary and do not contain any information or guidance related to coding or payment.

The CMS website offers a searchable database of LCDs by contractor (FI, carrier, and MAC) and contractor number. Once the specific contractor LCDs are accessed, the LCDs can be sorted by LCD ID, LCD Title, Effective Date, Revision Effective Date, LCD End Date, and Last Updated (Date).

The Resident Assessment Instrument User's Manual

Within all the administrative and clinical rules and regulations, there are more specific manuals, such as the *Resident Assessment Instrument (RAI) User's Manual*. This manual tells us in detail how to assess a resident, in ways that none of the aforementioned resources remotely touch on. October 1, 2010, brought about a significant change in the way residents in a SNF are assessed. As a result of this change, the *RAI User's Manual* was completely redone and offers guidance to SNFs on how to correctly and effectively assess a resident through the gathering and inputting of resident information into the minimum data set (MDS). The MDS is a clinical assessment tool required under federal mandate for all residents in either a Medicare- or Medicaid-covered stay in a nursing home.

Court cases

Finally, there are court cases, which serve as precedents for various issues. These cases typically involve reimbursement issues. To further complicate matters, not all court precedents make it into the manuals, transmittals, and so forth.

Summary

So there you have it: The Social Security Act, the *Federal Register*, Title *42 CFR*, manuals, program transmittals, LCDs, NCDs, the *RAI User's Manual*, and court precedents can all be valuable resources when determining skilled services.

The significance of discussing each of these resources is to show that not all issues related to skilled services can be addressed by a single resource. Sometimes you must use several resources in order to address some of the more complex issues.

The Online CMS Manual: IOM

Now that we have identified the sources of Medicare authority, it is time to focus on sections that will serve as valuable resources when making the determination of skilled services in a long-term care setting. When you are through with this section, you will be able to apply critical thinking to the situations you encounter in your own facility. The streamlined CMS manuals allow "one-stop shopping" to find the correct guidance for skilling a resident. Figure 1.2 outlines the Medicare Manual's table of contents, with which you should be somewhat familiar already.

We will focus on the main topics of each section that you will refer to often to support making skilled coverage decisions. All of these topics will be discussed in greater detail as you move through *Long-Term Care Skilled Services: Applying Medicare's Rules to Clinical Practice*, but this will provide you with some of the background information to begin asserting the role of decision-maker for skilled services in long-term care.

Although a majority of focus will be on Publication 100-02 (see Figure 1.3) because it contains the rules for skilling residents under Medicare, we will touch on other publications in the IOM that will serve as valuable information throughout the skilled care decision-making process. Within Publication 100-02, there are several chapters where the relationship between skilled service, eligibility, benefit periods, and payment is addressed.

FIGURE
1.2

CMS manual system: Table of contents

Publication #	Title
Pub. 100	Introduction
Pub. 100-01	*Medicare General Information, Eligibility, and Entitlement Manual*
Pub. 100-02	*Medicare Benefit Policy Manual*
Pub. 100-03	*Medicare National Coverage Determinations (NCD) Manual*
Pub. 100-04	*Medicare Claims Processing Manual*
Pub. 100-05	*Medicare Secondary Payer Manual*
Pub. 100-06	*Medicare Financial Management Manual*
Pub. 100-07	*State Operations Manual*
Pub. 100-08	*Medicare Program Integrity Manual*
Pub. 100-09	*Medicare Contractor Beneficiary and Provider Communications Manual*
Pub. 100-10	*Quality Improvement Organization Manual*
Pub. 100-11	*Reserved*
Pub. 100-12	*State Medicaid Manual (The new manual is under development. Please continue to use the paper-based manual to make your selection.)*
Pub. 100-13	*Medicaid State Children's Health Insurance Program (under development)*
Pub. 100-14	*Medicare ESRD Network Organizations Manual*
Pub. 100-15	*State Buy-In Manual*
Pub. 100-16	*Medicare Managed Care Manual*
Pub. 100-17	*CMS/Business Partners Systems Security Manual*
Pub. 100-18	*Reserved*
Pub. 100-19	*Demonstrations*
Pub. 100-20	*One-Time Notification*
Pub. 100-21	*Recurring Update Notification*
Pub. 100-22	*Medicare Quality Reporting Incentive Programs Manual*
Pub. 100-24	*State Buy-In Manual*

FIGURE

1.3

Pub. 100-02 *Medicare Benefit Policy Manual* chapters

CHAPTER	TITLE	FILE DOWNLOAD NAME
1	Inpatient Hospital Services	bp102c01.pdf
2	Inpatient Psychiatric Hospital Services	bp102c02.pdf
3	Duration of Covered Inpatient Services	bp102c03.pdf
4	Inpatient Psychiatric Benefit Days Reduction & Lifetime Limitation	bp102c04.pdf
5	Lifetime Reserve Days	bp102c05.pdf
6	Hospital Services Covered Under Part B	bp102c06.pdf
7	Home Health Services	bp102c07.pdf
8	Coverage of Extended Care (SNF) Services Under Hospital Insurance	bp102c08.pdf
9	Coverage of Hospice Services Under Hospital Insurance	bp102c09.pdf
10	Ambulance Services	bp102c10.pdf
11	End Stage Renal Disease (ESRD)	bp102c11.pdf
12	Comprehensive Outpatient Rehabilitation Facility (CORF) Coverage	bp102c12.pdf
13	Rural Health Clinic (RHC) & Federally Qualified Health Center (FQHC) Services	bp102c13.pdf
14	Medical Devices	bp102c14.pdf
15	Covered Medical & Other Health Services	bp102c15.pdf
16	General Exclusions From Coverage	bp102c16.pdf

FIGURE

1.4
Medicare Benefit Policy Manual

Chapter 8—Coverage of Extended Care (SNF) Services Under Hospital Insurance

10—Requirements - General

10.1—Medicare SNF PPS Overview

10.2—Medicare SNF Coverage Guidelines Under PPS

10.3—Hospital Providers of Extended Care Services

20—Prior Hospitalization and Transfer Requirements

20.1—Three-Day Prior Hospitalization

20.1.1—Three-Day Prior Hospitalization - Foreign Hospital

20.2—Thirty-Day Transfer

20.2.1—General

20.2.2—Medical Appropriateness Exception

20.2.2.1—Medical Needs Are Predictable

20.2.2.2—Medical Needs Are Not Predictable

20.2.2.3—SNF Stay Prior to Beginning of Deferred Covered Treatment

20.2.2.4—Effect of Delay in Initiation of Deferred Care

20.2.2.5—Effect on Spell of Illness

20.2.3—Readmission to a SNF

20.3—Payment Bans

20.3.1—Payment Bans on New Admissions

20.3.1.1—Beneficiary Notification

20.3.1.2—Readmissions and Transfers

20.3.1.3—Sanctions Lifted: Procedures for Beneficiaries Admitted During the Sanction Period

20.3.1.4—Payment Under Part B During a Payment Ban on New Admissions

20.3.1.5—Impact of Consolidated Billing Requirements

20.3.1.6—Impact on Spell of Illness

| FIGURE 1.4 | *Medicare Benefit Policy Manual* (cont.) |

30—Skilled Nursing Facility Level of Care - General

30.1—Administrative Level of Care Presumption

30.2—Skilled Nursing and Skilled Rehabilitation Services

30.2.1—Skilled Services Defined

30.2.2—Principles for Determining Whether a Service is Skilled

30.2.3—Specific Examples of Some Skilled Nursing or Skilled Rehabilitation Services

30.2.3.1—Management and Evaluation of a Patient Care Plan

30.2.3.2—Observation and Assessment of Patient's Condition

30.2.3.3—Teaching and Training Activities

30.2.4—Questionable Situations

30.3—Direct Skilled Nursing Services to Patients

30.4—Direct Skilled Rehabilitation Services to Patients

30.4.1—Skilled Physical Therapy

30.4.1.1—General

30.4.1.2—Application of Guidelines

30.4.2—Speech-Language Pathology

30.4.3—Occupational Therapy

30.5—Nonskilled Supportive or Personal Care Services

30.6—Daily Skilled Services Defined

30.7—Services Provided on an Inpatient Basis as a "Practical Matter"

30.7.1—The Availability of Alternative Facilities or Services

30.7.2—Whether Available Alternatives Are More Economical in the Individual Case

30.7.3—Whether the Patient's Physical Condition Would Permit Utilization of an Available, More Economical Care Alternative

40—Physician Certification and Recertification for Extended Care Services

40.1—Who May Sign the Certification or Recertification for Extended Care Services

| FIGURE 1.4 | *Medicare Benefit Policy Manual* (cont.) |

50—Covered Extended Care Services

50.1—Nursing Care Provided by or Under the Supervision of a Registered Professional Nurse

50.2—Bed and Board in Semi-Private Accommodations Furnished in Connection With Nursing Care

50.3—Physical Therapy, Speech-Language Pathology and Occupational Therapy Furnished by the Skilled Nursing Facility or by Others Under Arrangements With the Facility and Under Its Supervision

50.4—Medical Social Services to Meet the Patient's Medically Related Social Needs

50.5—Drugs and Biologicals

50.6—Supplies, Appliances, and Equipment

50.7—Medical Service of an Intern or Resident-in-Training

50.8—Other Services

50.8.1—General

50.8.2—Respiratory Therapy

60—Covered Extended Care Days

70—Medical and Other Health Services Furnished to SNF Patients

70.1—Diagnostic Services and Radiological Therapy

70.2—Ambulance Service

70.3—Inpatient Physical Therapy, Occupational Therapy, and Speech-Language Pathology Services

70.4—Services Furnished Under Arrangements With Providers

Note that Chapter 8 of Pub. 100-2 will be our primary avenue for determining whether a resident is skilled. As you read Chapter 8, you will see the various subsections that address specific issues. (see Figure 1.4). Think of the sections of Chapter 8 as providing the "answers to the test."

Figure 1.5 gives you a bird's-eye view of the rules, regulations, and resources available to you.

FIGURE 1.5	Rules, regulations, and resources tip sheet

Social Security Act	Enacted during the mid-1930s and amended during the mid-1960s to include the Medicare program. Several amendments and statutes have been introduced since. Updated in 1965 to include Medicare and Medicaid programs, commonly referred to as Title 18 and Title 19, respectively.
Omnibus Reconciliation Act of 1987	Demanded completion of the MDS to encourage skilled nursing facilities to assist residents in attaining and maintaining their highest level of function.
Balanced Budget Act of 1997	Initiated the prospective payment system (PPS) and consolidated billing for skilled nursing facilities. Also introduced the Medicare+Choice Program options for coverage.
Medicare, Medicaid and SCHIP Balanced Budget Refinement Act of 1999	Significant reimbursement impact to skilled nursing facility payments.
Medicare, Medicaid and SCHIP Benefits Improvement and Protection Act of 2000	Removal of market basket adjustment to skilled nursing facility payments, updates to Medicare+Choice regulations, consolidated billing refinements, and the Medicare Appeals Process.
Medicare Prescription Drug, Improvement and Modernization Act	Introduced the prescription drug benefit and entitlement referred to as Medicare Part D, changed name of Medicare+Choice to Medicare Advantage, and introduced the Medicare Administrative Contractor (MAC).
Federal Register	Updated continuously, related to new laws, proposed and changed rules and regulations.
Code of Federal Regulations 42 (42 CFR)	One source for anything related to public health.

FIGURE 1.5	Rules, regulations, and resources tip sheet (cont.)

Internet-Only Manuals (IOM)	Streamlined, updated, and consolidated versions of CMS' various program instructions into an electronic Web-based manual system for all users.
Program transmittals	CMS mandates, which are issued to intermediaries, carriers, and providers.
Medicare Learning Network (MLN) Articles	CMS published articles intended to provide practical operational information about the Medicare program.
National coverage determinations (NCDs)	Interpretations of federal rules, regulations, program transmittals, etc., for intermediaries, carriers, MACs, and providers.
Local coverage determinations (LCDs)	Intermediary, carrier, and MAC policies based on their interpretations of CMS' rules and regulations.
Resident Assessment Instrument (RAI) User's Manual	Instructions for assessing residents in nursing facilities using the MDS.
Publication 100-2, Chapter 8	Explains skilled service, skilled need, and skilled coverage.

FIGURE 1.6	Road map to Chapter 8

Internet-Only Manuals (IOMs)

↓

Publications
100 through 100-24

↓

Publication 100-2
Medicare Benefits Policy Manual

↓

CHAPTER 8
Coverage of Extended Care (SNF) Service Under Hospital Insurance (Part A)
Sections 10 through 70.4

Source: www.cms.hhs.gov/manuals.

Figure 1.6 is a flowchart that gives you a sense of how Chapter 8 evolved.

The layout of this book will mirror Chapter 8 of Publication 100-02 with added tips sheets, quick reference guides, case studies, and enhanced sections reviewing the MDS 3.0 in detail, focusing on both clinical and therapy needs.

As outlined by Figure 1.4, Chapter 8 of Publication 100-02 is broken out as follows:

- Section 10—Requirements – General

- Section 20—Prior Hospitalization and Transfer Requirements

- Section 30—Skilled Nursing Facility Level of Care – General

- Section 40—Physician Certification and Recertification for Extended Care Services

- Section 50—Covered Extended Care Services

- Section 60—Covered Extended Care Days

- Section 70—Medical and Other Health Services Furnished to SNF Patients

Once we get into Chapter 8, we will begin with Section 10, which will review the requirements of being classified as a SNF. Section 20 will highlight the technical eligibility requirements of coverage in a SNF; the transfer rules, windows, and exceptions; benefit periods; and how enrollment in other programs can impact coverage under traditional Medicare.

Then, Section 30 will allow us to start dissecting the world of skilled units. This section covers the following issues:

- Admission criteria

- The MDS and how it triggers a resource utilization group (RUG) score

- Definitions of skilled services

- Examples of skilled services

- Management and evaluation of the care plan

- Observation and assessment of the resident

- Questionable situations

- Direct nursing services to residents

- Direct rehabilitation services to skilled residents

- Nonskilled supportive services

- Defining daily skilled services

- Inpatient services versus alternative services

Section 40 will cover the requirements for a physician to certify and recertify skilled services in a SNF. Section 50 will identify the actual services that are required to be provided in a SNF under Medicare Part A and Part B. Finally, Sections 60 and 70 will outline what is considered a covered day and what other services are included in the SNF benefit.

Simple as that! You now know where to locate the resources and guidance for making decisions related to admitting and covering residents under Medicare in a SNF. The next several chapters will provide additional details, case studies, and additional information to make the process of skilling residents under Medicare in a SNF a very streamlined process.

Hierarchy of Oversight

CMS

CMS is a branch of the U.S. Department of Health and Human Services (HHS). CMS is the federal agency that administers the Medicare program and monitors the Medicaid programs offered by each state.

The following statements outline the mission, vision, and strategic action plan objectives of CMS:

- CMS' mission:

  - To ensure effective, up-to-date healthcare coverage and to promote quality care for beneficiaries

- CMS' vision:

  - To achieve a transformed and modernized healthcare system

  - CMS will accomplish this mission by continuing to transform and modernize America's healthcare system

- CMS' strategic action plan goals include the following:

  - Skilled, committed, and highly motivated workforce

  - Accurate and predictable payments

  - High-value healthcare

  - Confident, informed consumers

  - Collaborative partnerships

FI-Carrier Model

The dictionary definition of fiscal is "of or relating to financial matters." The dictionary definition of an intermediary is "a mediator or go-between." That being said, a fiscal intermediary, or an FI, is a mediator of financial matters. From a Medicare perspective, an FI is a private company with a Medicare contract to accept, process, pay, and review Medicare Part A claims and some Medicare Part B claims (depending on the provider type).

A Medicare carrier is similar to an FI in that they also accept, process, pay, and review Medicare claims, but only Medicare Part B claims (depending on the provider type), not Medicare Part A claims.

CMS is currently in the process of changing the current structure of the FI-Carrier, and converting all providers to a MAC. The duties and roles of the FIs and carriers will be absorbed by each individual MAC, with additional duties and responsibilities added.

MAC

As a component of the Medicare Modernization Act of 2003, CMS was required to convert the current provider oversight model of FIs and carriers that processed claims for different providers and either Medicare Part A or Part B. The new MAC model will allow one entity to process all Medicare Part A and Medicare Part B claims for fee-for-service claims (see Figure 1.7).

FIGURE
1.7

A/B MAC jurisdiction map

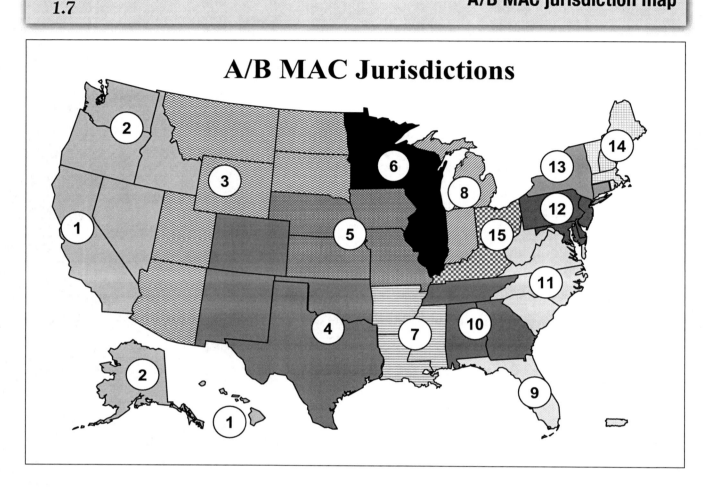

A/B MAC Jurisdictions

According to CMS,

[They] designed the new MAC jurisdictions to balance the allocation of workloads, promote competition, account for integration of claims processing activities, and mitigate the risk to the Medicare program during the transition to the new contractors. The new jurisdictions reasonably balance the number of fee-for-service beneficiaries and providers. These jurisdictions will be substantially more alike in size than the existing fiscal intermediary and carrier jurisdictions, and they will promote much greater efficiency in processing Medicare's billion claims a year.

The initial implementation to phase out fiscal intermediaries and carriers began in 2005 and will continue through 2011. CMS highlighted the following expected outcomes from the transition to the MAC model:

- Improved beneficiary services

  - Most beneficiaries will have their claims processed by only one contractor, reducing the number of separate explanation of benefits statements a beneficiary will receive and need to organize

  - A/B MACs will be required to develop an integrated and consistent approach to medical coverage across its service area, which benefits both beneficiaries and providers

  - Beneficiaries will be able to have their questions on claims answered by calling 1-800-MEDICARE, their single point of contact

- Improved provider services

  - A simplified interface with a single MAC for Part A and Part B processing and other services will benefit providers

  - Competition will encourage MACs to deliver better service to providers

  - Requiring MACs to focus on financial management will result in more accurate claims payments and greater consistency in payment decisions

Office of Inspector General

The mission of the Office of Inspector General (OIG) is:

[T]o protect the integrity of Department of Health and Human Services (HHS) programs, as well as the health and welfare of the beneficiaries of those programs. The OIG has a responsibility to report both to the Secretary and to the Congress program and management problems and recommendations to correct them. The OIG's duties are carried out through a nationwide network of audits, investigations, inspections and other mission-related functions performed by OIG components.

In March 2000, the OIG published the *Compliance Program Guidance for Nursing Facilities*. According to the OIG, "The creation of compliance program guidance is a major initiative of the OIG in its effort to engage the private healthcare community in combating fraud and abuse." In late 1998, the OIG published a public notice to solicit information and recommendations for developing compliance programs and guidance for skilled nursing facilities. The information submitted along with that request was carefully reviewed along with other information previously published by the OIG to develop the compliance guidance for SNFs and also the OIG *Supplemental Compliance Program Guidance for Nursing Facilities*, published in September 2008. The following elements of an effective compliance program were published in *65 FR 14289*, in March 16, 2000:

- Implementing written policies, procedures, and standards of conduct

- Designating a compliance officer and compliance committee

- Conducting effective training and education

- Developing effective lines of communication

- Enforcing standards through well-publicized disciplinary guidelines

- Conducting internal monitoring and auditing

- Responding promptly to detected offenses and developing corrective action

In addition to the monitoring of compliance, the OIG is also responsible for the following:

- Safe harbor regulations and anti-kickback statues

- Medicare and Medicaid fraud control

- Provider-specific work plans that identify target areas of review on an annual basis

Government Accounting Office

The Government Accounting Office (GAO) investigates how the federal government, including CMS, spends taxpayer dollars. They are an independent agency that is engaged for special reviews, reports, and projects as directed by Congress. Specifically, some of the duties of the GAO include the following:

- Auditing agency operations to determine whether federal funds are being spent efficiently and effectively

- Investigating allegations of illegal and improper activities

- Reporting on how well government programs and policies are meeting their objectives

- Performing policy analyses and outlining options for congressional consideration

- Issuing legal decisions and opinions, such as bid protest rulings and reports on agency rules

CHAPTER 2

Technical Eligibility for Skilled Services in Long-Term Care

Before we can begin to look at whether the care to be delivered in the skilled nursing facility (SNF) will meet the requirements, we need to be sure that the potential resident has met the technical criteria for Medicare Part A services in the SNF. Therefore, we will review the following questions in detail:

- Who is generally eligible for Medicare benefits?

- Are the benefits verified?

- Are the transfer requirements met?

- Which days are available in the current benefit period?

- Is care a continuation of care related to reason for hospitalization?

Who Is Generally Eligible for Medicare Benefits?

An individual can be eligible for Medicare benefits if the individual falls under any of the following categories:

- Is age 65 and has paid at least 40 quarters into the Medicare program during his or her lifetime

- Is under age 65, is disabled, and has met the Medicare criteria for eligibility for disabled individuals

- Has been diagnosed with end stage renal disease (ESRD) at any age

Individuals age 65 and older who have paid the 40 quarters into the Medicare program become eligible on day 1 of the month in which they turn 65 and pay nothing for coverage under Medicare Part A. For Medicare Part B, every beneficiary pays a monthly premium; the amount of the monthly premium depends on entitlement, income level, and whether enrollment was delayed. For example, if an individual turns 65 on June 27, Medicare eligibility will begin on June 1. If any individual only paid between 30–39 quarters into the Medicare program, the Medicare benefit can be purchased at a reduced rate.

Disabled individuals under age 65 who have met the criteria for disability benefits under Social Security can also be entitled to Medicare as a result of that disability status. There is generally a two-year waiting period to qualify for Medicare benefits in this case. Individuals who have been diagnosed with ESRD (i.e., permanent kidney failure requiring either a kidney transplant or dialysis) are also eligible.

Are the Benefits Verified?

Possession of a Medicare card does not guarantee benefits. Possession of a Medicare card can only tell you that a beneficiary was, at one time, entitled to Medicare benefits. There are several other programs and factors that can impact current eligibility.

All SNF providers who have access to the Medicare Direct Data Entry (DDE) System have access to what is commonly referred to as the Common Working File (CWF). The CWF is updated as providers add bills for services, as updates are communicated by Social Security, or as coverage details are updated by other programs such as managed care providers, home health, and hospice providers.

The CWF has a minimum of 11 screens of data detailing the current benefits available to the beneficiary being queried. Additional screens from 12 and up detail coverage in other programs such as liability policies, employee group health plans, etc., that are primary to Medicare; more will be discussed on that primary coverage to Medicare later in this section. Although the CWF is a great place to obtain up-to-date information on a beneficiary's current benefit, it is important to note that the CWF is updated as providers add bills for services. That said, often the count of days available in the current benefit period can be lagging due to the billing practices of the last provider to render services. Staff accessing the CWF must keep in mind that information can have anywhere from a 30–60 day delay, depending on provider claim processing, etc.

The CWF is updated as providers bill for services. It is important to note that the CWF is updated as providers submit claims for services. The CWF offers the following information, related to eligibility, for providers to review:

- Date of entitlement to Medicare Part A and Medicare Part B benefits

- Date of termination of Medicare Part A and Medicare Part B benefits

- Days available in both the current and prior benefit periods

- Enrollment in a health maintenance organization (HMO), status of current and prior home health episodes, election of the Medicare hospice benefit, and other insurance information that is primary to Medicare.

Date of entitlement indicates the month, day, and year the individual was originally entitled to the Medicare benefit. Date of termination indicates the day, month, and year the beneficiary's entitlement in the Medicare program was terminated. Benefits can be terminated for any of the following reasons:

- An individual who purchases the Medicare Part A benefit, possibly due to not meeting the 40 quarter requirement, who stops paying for the benefit

- As previously noted, every beneficiary pays a monthly premium for the Medicare Part B benefit and this benefit can also be terminated for failure to pay

How does the use of home health services or hospice election affect traditional Medicare?

The Medicare home health benefit also qualifies as an inpatient benefit, similar to the Medicare SNF benefit. A beneficiary using the home health benefit is essentially an inpatient in his or her own home. The home health benefit has specific criteria regarding a beneficiary's "homebound status" that is required to be met before Medicare home health services can be used. That said, only one inpatient benefit can be used at a time; Medicare home health and Medicare SNF benefits cannot be used for the same resident for the same period of time.

When a resident elects the hospice benefit, it is elected in lieu of traditional Medicare. The hospice benefit is available to those individuals deemed by a physician to have a terminal illness. Similar to the home health benefit, the hospital benefit also qualifies as an inpatient benefit. One difference, though, is that a beneficiary can receive hospice services not only in the home, but also in a SNF or an inpatient hospice unit. Confused? Let me throw another wrinkle in there. It is possible for Medicare to reimburse both hospice and a SNF for the same beneficiary for the same dates of service. This is only possible when the reason for treatment in the SNF is completely unrelated to the diagnosis for hospice. This should not happen very often, but is a possibility and will require cohesive documentation on both the SNF and hospice medical records to illustrate that the reasons for the treatment and diagnosis are completely unrelated. The SNF would be required to show special coding on the claim to indicate that the overlap with hospice election is allowable. However, providers should be cautioned to verify that documentation exists prior to treatment under both programs.

With that said, Medicare Part A, often referred to as the inpatient benefit, cannot cover the same resident under more than one of the following programs at the same time (unless it is the specific hospice situation previously noted):

- Inpatient hospital

- SNF

- Hospice

- Home health

How does enrollment in other programs affect traditional Medicare?

There are also potential areas for coverage that is primary to traditional Medicare in the case of policies known as Medicare Replacement plans such as HMO, preferred provider organization (PPO), or private-fee-for-service (PFFS). There is also the potential for Medicare to be secondary to the following coverage:

- Employee group health plans (EGHP)

- Workers' compensation

- No-fault policies

- Liability policies

- Auto medical expense policies

In the case of Medicare replacement plans, the beneficiary's benefits are assigned to the plan and only the plan can bill Medicare for services. In most cases, a contract or preauthorization for treatment must be obtained before the SNF can treat the resident and be reimbursed for services. SNF claims submitted to Medicare for residents enrolled in a Medicare replacement plan will be denied for primary coverage under the Medicare replacement policy.

For Medicare secondary policies—as bulleted previously—these plans do not take the place of Medicare as do Medicare replacement plans, but are required to be billed primary before Medicare can be billed secondary. These are often listed on screens 12 and above on the CWF. Unlike Medicare replacement policies, Medicare will make secondary payment for any balance due on a claim billed to one of the primary payers noted previously, such as an auto expense policy. However, special calculations need to be made to determine if any balance will be paid by Medicare after the primary insurance has made payment. Per Section 40.8.2 of Publication 100-05, Chapter 5:

The amount of secondary benefits payable to providers is the lowest of the following:

- *The gross amount payable by Medicare ... minus the applicable deductible and/or coinsurance amount; or,*

- *The gross amount payable by Medicare minus the amount paid by the primary payer for Medicare covered services; or,*

- *The provider's charges (or an amount less than the charges that the provider is obligated to accept as payment in full), minus the amount paid by the primary payer for Medicare covered services; or*

- *The provider's charges (or an amount less than the charges that the provider is obligated to accept in full), minus the applicable Medicare deductible and/or coinsurance amounts.*

There are additional requirements that will need to be reviewed in relation to accepting payment as payment in full if the provider has a preferred provider agreement; for example, in the case of an EGHP or if there are resident deductibles and/or copayments involved, the provider may not be able to bill any balance to Medicare. Please review Chapter 5 of Publication 100-05 for additional calculation details and other considerations when billing Medicare as a secondary payer.

FIGURE
2.1

Common working file access

```
MAP1751                    M E D I C A R E A O N L I N E S Y S T E M
SC                              ELIGIBILITY DETAIL INQUIRY

HIC                 CURR XREF HIC                    PREV XREF HIC
TRANSFER HIC                        C-IND        LTR DAYS
LN                       FN              MI      SEX
DOB            DOD
ADDR                            CITY
ST      ZIP

                          CURRENT ENTITLEMENT
PART A EFF DT            TERM DT          PART B EFF DT        TERM DT

   CURRENT              BENEFIT PERIOD DATA
FRST BILL DT           LST BILL DT     HSP FULL DAYS          HSP PART DAYS
SNF FULL DAYS       SNF PART DAYS    INP DED REMAIN           BLD DED PNTS

                            PSYCHIATRIC
PSY DAYS REMAIN      PRE PHY DAYS USED      PSY DIS DT        INTRM DT IND

PRESS PF3-EXIT PF8-NEXT PAGE
```

Shaded areas denote required fields to access beneficiary information

HIC	Beneficiary's Health Insurance Claim Number
CURR XREF HIC	If the HIC number has changed for the beneficiary, this field represents the most recent number.
PREV XREF HIC	This field is no longer in use.
TRANSFER HIC	This field is no longer in use.
C-IND Century indicator	This field represents a one position code identifying if the beneficiary's date of birth is in the 18th or 19th century. Valid values are: 8 = 1800s 9 = 1900s
LTR DAYS	Lifetime reserve days remaining.

    Long-Term Care Skilled Services

FIGURE
2.1

Common working file access (cont.)

LN	Beneficiary's last name.
FN	Beneficiary's first name.
MI	Beneficiary's middle initial.
SEX	Beneficiary's sex.
DOB	Beneficiary's date of birth. Must be entered in MMDDYYYY format.
DOD	Beneficiary's date of death.
ADDR	Beneficiary's street address.
CITY	Beneficiary's city of residence.
ST	Beneficiary's state of residence.
ZIP	Zip code for state of residence.
PART A EFF DT	Date beneficiary's Medicare Part A benefits become effective.
TERM DT	Date beneficiary's Medicare Part A benefits were terminated.
PART B EFF DT	Date beneficiary's Medicare Part B benefits became effective.
TERM DT	Date beneficiary's Medicare Part B benefits were terminated.
FRST BILL DT	Beginning date of benefit period.
LST BILL DT	Ending date of benefit period.
HSP FULL DAYS	Hospital full days remaining.
HSP PART DAYS	Hospital co-insurance days remaining.
SNF FULL DAYS	Skilled nursing facility full days remaining.
SNF PART DAYS	Skilled nursing facility partial days remaining.
INP DED REMAIN	Amount of Medicare Part A inpatient deductible, beneficiary must still pay.
BLD DED PNTS	Number of blood deductible pints remaining to be met.
PSYCHIATRIC PSY DAYS REMAIN	Number of psychiatric days remaining.
PRE PHY DYS USED	Number of pre-entitlement psychiatric days the beneficiary has used.
PSY DIS DT	Date beneficiary was discharged from a level of care.
INTRM DT IND	Code that indicates an interim date for psychiatric services. Valid values are: Y = Date is through date of interim bill/utilization day N = Discharge date/not a utilization day

Are the Transfer Requirements Met?

With regard to transfer requirements to use Medicare Part A benefits in a SNF, Section 20 of Publication 100-02, Chapter 8 states:

In order to qualify for post-hospital extended care services, the individual must have been an inpatient of a hospital for a medically necessary stay of at least three consecutive calendar days. In addition, effective December 5, 1980, the individual must have been transferred to a participating SNF within 30 days after discharge from the hospital.

It is further defined in that same reference that the discharge from the hospital must have occurred on or after the first day of the month in which the beneficiary turned 65. The three days must have been consecutive, and time spent in an observation stay or in the emergency room do not count toward this requirement. The three days will only count for this requirement if the beneficiary was admitted as an inpatient of the hospital for three consecutive midnights; the day of admission counts toward this requirement, but the day of discharge does not.

It is also important to understand what types of institutions qualify as a hospital for this purpose. The hospital must be either a Medicare-participating hospital or an institution that meets at least the conditions of participation for an emergency services hospital (see Publication 100-01, *Medicare General Information, Eligibility, and Entitlement*, Chapter 5, §20.2, for definition of an emergency services hospital). A nonparticipating psychiatric hospital need not meet the special requirements applicable to psychiatric hospitals. Stays in religious nonmedical healthcare institutions (see Publication 100-01, *Medicare General Information, Eligibility, and Entitlement*, Chapter 5, §40, for definition of Religious Nonmedical Health Care Institution [RNHCI]) are excluded for the purpose of satisfying the three-day period of hospitalization. Publication 100-01, *Medicare General Information, Eligibility, and Entitlement*, Chapter 5, §20.2 defines an emergency hospital as follows:

An emergency services hospital is a nonparticipating hospital which meets the requirements of the law's definition of a "hospital" relating to full-time nursing services and licensure under State or applicable local law. (A Federal hospital need not be licensed under State or local licensing laws to meet the definition of emergency hospital.) In addition, the hospital must be primarily engaged in providing, under the supervision of doctors of medicine or osteopathy, services of the type that §20.1 describes in defining the term hospital, and must not be primarily engaged in providing skilled nursing care and related services for patients who require medical or nursing care. Psychiatric hospitals that meet these requirements can qualify as emergency hospitals.

It is equally important to note that although a qualifying stay in a psychiatric hospital will meet this requirement, there is an additional requirement related to continuing the care received in the hospital that may preclude a SNF from covering a resident in the SNF under Medicare in such instances.

Now it is possible for a beneficiary to qualify for Medicare Part A benefits in a SNF and not have a three-day hospital stay within the last 30 calendar days.

You will note in the first reference to Section 20 of Publication 100-02, Chapter 8, it is noted that the transfer to the SNF must have been within 30 days of discharge from the hospital. A beneficiary may be readmitted to the original or other SNF within 30 days of discharge from the initial SNF stay as well. The transfer requirement of 30 days is either from the time of hospital discharge or Medicare Part A SNF stay following that hospitalization.

Medical appropriateness exception

There are some situations where a delay of more than 30 days between hospital discharge and SNF admission are allowable; this provision is called the *Medical Appropriateness Exception* and is detailed in Section 20.2.2 of Publication 100-02, Chapter 8.

An elapsed period of more than 30 days is permitted for SNF admissions when the patient's condition makes it medically inappropriate to begin an active course of treatment in a SNF immediately after hospital discharge, and it is medically predictable at the time of the hospital discharge that he or she will require covered care within a predetermined period of time. The fact that a patient enters a SNF immediately upon discharge from a hospital, for either covered or noncovered care, does not necessarily negate coverage at a later date, assuming the subsequent covered care was medically predictable.

So, this statement then brings up the following question: What makes care "medically predictable?" It is important to note that the overall purpose of the SNF benefit is to cover short-term care to continue services received in the hospital; this, in part, points to the 30-day transfer window to be able to relate the SNF care back to the hospitalization. Section 20.2.2.1 of the same publication notes the following:

Since the exception is intended to apply only where the SNF care constitutes a continuation of care provided in the hospital, it is applicable only where, under accepted medical practice, the established pattern of treatment for a particular condition indicates that a covered level of SNF care will be required within a predeterminable time frame. Accordingly, to qualify for this exception it must be medically predictable at the time of hospital discharge that a covered level of SNF care will be required within a predictable period of time for the treatment of a condition for which hospital care was received and the patient must begin receiving such care within that time frame.

The regulation goes on to provide the following example situation of medical appropriateness and medical predictability:

An example of the type of care for which this provision was designed is care for a person with a hip fracture. Under the established pattern of treatment of hip fractures it is known that skilled therapy services will be required subsequent to hospital care, and that they can normally begin within four to six weeks after hospital discharge, when weight bearing can be tolerated. Under the exception to the 30-day rule, the admission of a patient with a hip fracture to a SNF within 4 to 6 weeks after hospital discharge for skilled care, which as a practical matter can only be provided on an inpatient basis by a SNF, would be considered a timely admission.

In short, in order to qualify under both provisions to delay a SNF admission for more than 30 days, the following criteria must be met:

- The beneficiary's condition requires a delay in treatment of more than 30 days that is predictable and documented by a physician prior to discharge from the qualifying hospital stay

- The predetermined time in which to delay treatment is also documented by the physician prior to discharge from the qualifying hospital stay

In instances where the care is not predictable at the time of hospital discharge, the *Centers for Medicare & Medicaid Services (CMS) Manual* simply states:

When a patient's medical needs and the course of treatment are not predictable at the time of hospital discharge because the exact pattern of care required and the time frame in which it will be required is dependent on the developing nature of the patient's condition, an admission to a SNF more than 30 days after discharge from the hospital is not justified under this exception to the 30-day rule.

Which Days Are Available in the Current Benefit Period?

Before we can take a look at whether the care to be received in the SNF is a necessary continuation of the reason for hospitalization or is a condition that arose during the hospitalization, we need to review and understand the nuances of SNF benefit periods. This information can be found in Publication 100-01, Chapter 3, Section 4.

Publication 100-1, General Eligibility Manual, Chapter 3, Section 10.4

Section 10.4 addresses the benefit period or "spell of illness" component—an integral component to understanding skilled care and its impact. It was revised in 2002 and there are specific rules that apply only to the SNF. Sometimes the level of care in the SNF is referred to as "extended care" in the regulations. The specific items to be reviewed include the following:

Section 10.4.1: Starting a Benefit Period

A benefit period begins with the first day on which a patient is furnished in an inpatient hospital or extended care services by a qualified provider in a month for which the patient is entitled to hospital insurance benefits. When the regulation refers to hospital insurance benefits, the Medicare Part A program is indicated.

Section 10.4.2: Ending a Benefit Period

A benefit period ends when a beneficiary has not been an inpatient of a SNF or when skilled services are no longer required or received for at least 60 consecutive days (counted from the day of discharge). Then there is a special note for SNFs: See Section 10.4.3.2, which follows, for determining the end of a benefit period when an individual remains in a SNF.

Section 10.4.3.2: SNF Stay and End of Benefit Period

This section defines a SNF for purposes of ending the benefit period and contains several examples that cover some of the more common situations encountered.

Section 10.4.4: Definition of Inpatient for Ending a Benefit Period (special for SNFs)

A different definition of inpatient applies in determining the end of a benefit period for a beneficiary in a SNF: A beneficiary is an inpatient in a SNF only if the beneficiary's care in the SNF meets certain skilled-level-of-care standards. The beneficiary must need and receive a skilled level of care while in the SNF. This means that in order to have been an inpatient while in a SNF, the beneficiary must have required and received skilled services on a daily basis, which could, as a practical matter, have been provided only in an SNF on an inpatient basis. If these provisions were not met during the prior SNF stay, the beneficiary was not an inpatient of the SNF for purposes of prolonging the benefit period.

There are seven presumptions listed in Chapter 3 regarding the beneficiary's care in a SNF rising to the level of skilled care. Another important issue discussed and worth noting here because many facilities may not be following this rule consistently is the fact that Medicare no-payment bills that a SNF submits result in Medicare program payment determinations (i.e., denials). Therefore, such no-payment bills trigger the appropriate presumptions. This also applies in any state where the Medicaid program uses no-payment bills that lead to Medicaid program payment determinations. If a SNF erroneously fails to submit a Medicare claim (albeit a no-pay claim) when Medicare rules require such submission, intermediaries request a SNF to submit one. Once the no-pay bill is submitted and denied, the applicable presumption (other than presumption 7) is triggered. If a patient is moving from a SNF level of care to a non-SNF level of care in a facility certified to provide SNF care, occurrence code 22 (date active care ended) is used to signify the beginning of the no-pay period on the bill and to trigger the appropriate presumptions.

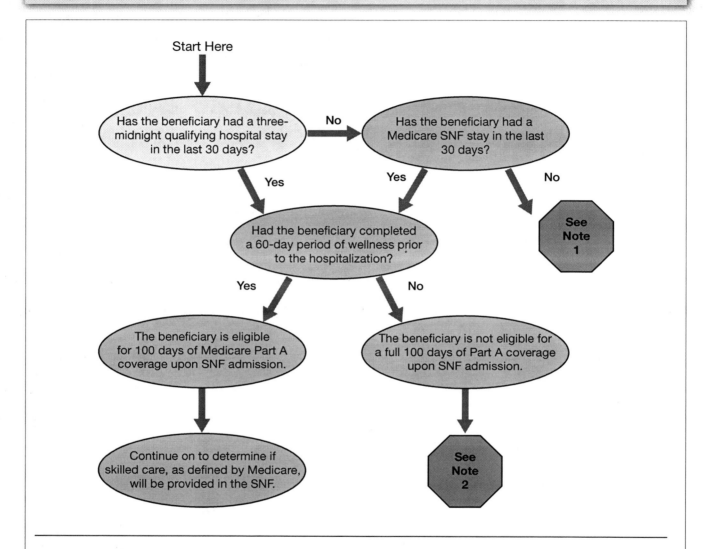

FIGURE
2.3

Benefit period decision-maker

Note 1: A resident must have a qualifying hospital stay or Medicare SNF stay within the last 30 days to use the Medicare Part A SNF benefit. If the resident does not meet one of these two criteria and was not using the Medical appropriateness exception for the delay in admission, the resident will not qualify.

Note 2: If the resident did not meet the requirement for a 60-day period of wellness, he or she will only be able to use the days remaining in the current benefit period. For example, if prior to the hospitalization or SNF discharge, the resident used 60 Medicare Part A SNF days, there will only be 40 days available for the current admission. If 75 Medicare Part A SNF days were used, there will be only 25 available for the current admission. Earning a new 100-day benefit period has nothing to do with a new diagnosis or diagnosis at all; it is strictly tied to that requirement for a 60-day period of wellness before a new 100-day period can be earned.

Is Care a Continuation of Care Related to the Reason for Hospitalization?

As previously discussed, SNF services are often referred to as extended care services due to the fact that they represent an extension of services received during the three-day qualifying hospital stay.

Per Section 10 of Publication 100-02, Chapter 8 states:

> [T]he beneficiary must require SNF care for a condition that was treated during the qualifying hospital stay, or for a condition that arose while in the SNF for treatment of a condition for which the beneficiary was previously treated in the hospital.

Before it can be determined if the care to be received is skilled in nature, the care must have a direct correlation back to the reason for hospitalization or to continue treatment for a condition that arose during the hospital stay. As a matter of principal, Medicare will only cover services that are to return a beneficiary back to his or her prior level of function. This sums up the requirement to correlate SNF treatment with a hospital admission.

How does a payment ban impact Medicare coverage in a SNF?

Section 20.3.1 of Publication 100-02, Chapter 8 defines this situation as such:

> Under the Social Security Act at §§1819(h) and 1919(h) and CMS' regulations at 42 CFR 488.417, CMS may impose a denial of payment for new admissions (DPNA) against a SNF when CMS finds that a facility is not in substantial compliance with requirements of participation. Further, the regulations require CMS to impose a DPNA when a SNF (1) fails to be in substantial compliance for three months after the last day of the survey identifying the noncompliance, or (2) is found to have provided substandard quality of care on the last three consecutive standard surveys. FIs are responsible for applying these payment sanctions to new SNF admissions resulting from adverse survey findings. The SNFs under a denial of payment sanction are still considered Medicare-participating providers.

When a DPNA has been imposed on a SNF, the SNF is not allowed to accept any new admissions during that time or bill Medicare for the stay. We will discuss the definition of a "new admission" shortly. But, for an individual that does qualify as a new admission, the SNF has the following choices:

1. Accept the resident and be the provider liable for the stay (the SNF will not receive reimbursement from Medicare or the beneficiary)

2. Notify the beneficiary of the DPNA in writing prior to admission and require the beneficiary to pay for the SNF care received during the DPNA

Special billing requirements apply to both situations noted and can be found in Section 50 of Publication 100-05, Chapter 6—*Medicare Claims Processing Manual.*

Criteria for beneficiary notification to accept payment from the beneficiary during a DPNA are very specific and are as follows:

1. It must be in writing

2. It must explain the reason sanctions were imposed

3. It must explain the beneficiary's liability for the cost of SNF services during the period the payment ban is in effect

4. It must explain that Medicare Part A benefits may be available if the beneficiary chooses a different Medicare-participating SNF that is not under sanction

If a SNF fails to provide such a notice, then the provider is considered liable for the beneficiary's stay.

In addition, the DPNA only applies to Medicare Part A services, not Medicare Part B services. Section 20.3.1.4 of the previously referenced manual states:

Facilities subject to a payment ban may continue to bill services for beneficiaries who are not in a Part A stay in the same way as any other SNF. However, services that would have been payable to the SNF as Part A benefits in the absence of a payment sanction must not be billed to either the FI [fiscal intermediary] or the carrier as Part B services.

What is considered a new admission?

Section 20.3.1 of Publication 100-02, Chapter 8 states:

> *Imposition of a payment ban on SNF new admissions is described in 42 CFR 488.401. In applying payment bans, refer to the following definition of "new admission" to a SNF contained in 42 CFR 488.401. [a] Resident who is admitted to the facility on or after the effective date of a denial of payment remedy and, if previously admitted, has been discharged before that effective date. Residents admitted before the effective date of the denial of payment, and taking temporary leave, are not considered new admissions, nor subject to the denial of payment.*

It is important to also note that the resident need not have been a Medicare resident prior to the temporary leave discharge to be exempt from being deemed a new admission. Their status as a resident prior to the payment ban is what needs to be reviewed, not the payer type prior to discharge.

Is there an impact to the benefit period?

Residents receiving skilled services under a DPNA are still deemed to have been provided skilled services, even though Medicare was not billed for such services. Therefore, any time either the provider accepts liability for the services or charges the beneficiary for the services (provided the notification criteria were met, as previously outlined), this would still count toward skilled care and would not count as part of a 60-day period of wellness needed to qualify for a new benefit period; and claims should be submitted as such.

CHAPTER 3

Meeting the Regulatory Guidelines for "Skilled" Services in a Skilled Nursing Facility

Now that we have determined that a resident meets the technical criteria for Medicare Part A coverage in a skilled nursing facility (SNF), we need to review whether the resident meets the definition of skilled services according to the regulatory requirements and the criteria for certification of those services.

Publication 100-02, *Medicare Benefit Policy Manual*, Chapter 8, Section 30

Section 30 thoroughly defines a skilled resident. These level-of-care requirements specify that the following four criteria must be met:

- *The patient requires skilled nursing services or skilled rehabilitation services (i.e., **services that must be performed by or under the supervision of professional or technical personnel** [see §30.2– 30.4]) are ordered by a physician and the services are rendered for a condition for which the patient received inpatient hospital services, or for a condition that arose while receiving care in a SNF for a condition for which he or she received inpatient hospital services;*

- *The patient requires these skilled services on a daily basis (see §30.6); and*

- *As a practical matter, considering economy and efficiency, the daily skilled services can be provided only on an inpatient basis in a SNF (see §30.7).*

- *The services must be reasonable and necessary for the treatment of a patient's illness or injury (i.e., be consistent with the nature and severity of the individual's illness or injury and the individual's particular medical needs, and be accepted standards of medical practice). The services must also be reasonable in terms of duration and quantity.*

This section of the manual goes on to stress that all of these components must be met before you can skill a resident.

Note the bolded words in the previous paragraph: SNF services "**must be performed by or under the supervision of professional or technical personnel**." Facilities frequently have a major misconception about this topic. An RN, physician, physical therapist (PT), occupational therapist (OT), or speech-language pathologist (SLP) must render skilled services. Notice, however, that Centers for Medicare & Medicaid Services (CMS) says these services must be performed under a licensed professional's supervision. A licensed professional is someone who holds a valid recognized license, such as a licensed vocational nurse, licensed practical nurse (LPN), RN, nurse practitioner (NP), physician's assistant, physician, PT, OT, SLP, or respiratory therapist.

Furthermore, "supervision" does not necessarily mean that the licensed professional has to be in direct sight of the persons giving care. For example, if a restorative aide is working with a resident or if nurses' aides are providing a two-person assist in a resident's room, the licensed professional does not have to be in the same room.

Section 30.2.1: Skilled services defined

Section 30.2.1 ("Skilled Nursing and Skilled Rehabilitation Services") provides definitions of "skilled nursing" and "skilled rehabilitation services." It stipulates that under a physician's order for services, a licensed professional (such as an RN, LPN, PT, OT, or SLP) must provide direct care or general supervision of care. "General supervision" is defined as "requiring initial direction and periodic inspection of the actual activity." The section further states, "The supervisor need not always be physically present."

Section 30.2.2: Determining whether services are skilled—criteria for determination

Section 30.2.2 ("Determining Whether a Service is Skilled") starts to look more closely at the criteria for assessing a skilled need. The regulation states, "The skilled service must be so inherently complex, that it can only be safely and effectively performed by a licensed, nonphysician, professional." It goes on to state that a condition that would not ordinarily require skilled services may still qualify for skilled care if there are "special medical complications." For example, a resident might have a plaster cast on a leg. A skilled service might exist if the resident requires traction adjustments for the leg, or if there is a preexisting skin condition that requires observation by a licensed nonphysician professional to observe for complications.

In addition, this section clarifies another misconception: A patient must show improvement or have the ability to improve in order to be admitted to a skilled unit. This assumption is incorrect, as illustrated by the section of the manual that states, "While a patient's particular medical condition is a valid factor in deciding if skilled services are needed or not, a patient's diagnosis or prognosis (restorative potential) should never be the sole factor in deciding that a service is not skilled."

To support this point, the manual offers four examples of residents who can be skilled but who do not necessarily demonstrate improvement or have the ability to demonstrate improvement.

- A resident who needs therapy that is not based on potential recovery but is based on whether the expertise of the therapist is needed could be considered skilled

- Although whirlpool baths are not considered skilled, when a PT intervenes for a resident because of the resident's circulatory deficiencies, desensitization, or open wounds, these types of treatments would be skilled

- A resident who has a variety of complications that by themselves would not qualify as skilled, but that as a whole need the involvement of daily skilled nursing to manage the total care plan could be considered skilled

- Turning a resident to avoid decubitus ulcers is not a skilled service in itself, but when issues arise with regard to a risk of improper body alignment, contractures, and deformities, with proper documentation, the resident could be considered skilled

A good lesson from this section is that in light of any individual service, skilled coverage may not be warranted. Rather, you must take into account the resident's total condition and then your skilled management of the services provided as the basis to determine whether you can skill a resident.

Section 30.2.3.1: Management and evaluation of a patient care plan

Per Section 30.2.3.1, titled "Management and Evaluation of a Patient Care Plan":

The development, management, and evaluation of a patient care plan, based on the physician's orders, constitute skilled nursing services when, in terms of the patient's physical or mental condition, these services require the involvement of skilled nursing personnel to meet the patient's medical needs, promote recovery, and ensure medical safety. However, the planning and management of a treatment plan that does not involve the furnishing of skilled services may not require skilled nursing personnel; e.g., a care plan for a patient with organic brain syndrome who requires only oral medication and a protective environment. The sum total of nonskilled services would only add up to the need for skilled management and evaluation when the condition of the beneficiary is such that there is an expectation that a change in condition is likely without that intervention.

Although we will discuss the minimum data set (MDS) later in this book, realize that the verbiage from Section 30.2.3.1 is an important piece of the puzzle when viewed in conjunction with resident assessments and the resident's total condition.

For instance, the example in Section 30.2.3.1 discusses a resident who suffers from several minor issues that, on the surface, could be treated by a less qualified but well-instructed staff member. However, the example is quick to point out that the instructed staff member may not have the expertise or training to recognize how the various services or treatments interact with one another and affect the overall picture. This lack of knowledge can lead to poor documentation and observation, which can negatively affect the resident. Thus, the knowledge of an RN, LPN, PT, OT, and/or SLP can be invaluable.

A similar example that Section 30.2.3.1 provides is a resident with pneumonia, chest congestion, a debilitating condition, and confusion. Once again, you need to look at the total care of the resident in order to determine who should provide care and whether you can skill that resident.

Section 30.2.3.2: Observation and assessment of a resident's condition

One of the many "urban legends" is that a resident can be skilled for five days, eight days, or 14 days to observe and assess his or her condition. This is simply not true. Nothing in the rules states that you need to skill a resident for observation and assessment for a certain number of days. Section 30.2.3.2 breaks this topic down into even further detail.

Observation and assessment are skilled services when the likelihood of change in a patient's condition requires skilled nursing or skilled rehabilitation personnel to identify and evaluate the patient's need for possible modification of treatment or initiation of additional medical procedures, until the patient's treatment regimen is essentially stabilized.

The manual does a good job of pointing out examples of observation and assessment, such as the following:

- Monitoring fluid levels

- Monitoring for decompensation

- Monitoring for adverse effects from medications

- Monitoring an adverse reaction to a surgical procedure

- Monitoring skin breakdown

These are just a few of many, many examples. Maybe the staff focuses on getting a resident's nutrition level back to where it needs to be after a spell of pneumonia. This may involve tube feeding, monitoring the resident's weight, and evaluating for any possible signs of dehydration. The skilled scenario possibilities are endless.

Section 30.2.3.3: Teaching and training activities

You may have heard that a facility can skill a resident for teaching and training activities, but facilities rarely use such avenues for skilling. The most prominent teaching and training activities include the following:

- Teaching self-administration of injectable medications or a complex range of medications

- Teaching a newly diagnosed diabetic to administer insulin injections, to prepare and follow a diabetic diet, and to observe foot-care precautions

- Teaching self-administration of medical gases to a resident

- Gait training and teaching of prosthesis care to a resident who has had a recent leg amputation

- Teaching residents how to care for a recent colostomy or ileostomy

- Teaching residents how to perform self-catheterization and self-administration of gastrostomy feedings

- Teaching residents how to care for and maintain central venous lines, such as Hickman catheters

- Teaching residents how to use and care for braces, splints, and orthotics and to perform any associated skin care

- Teaching residents the proper care of any specialized dressings or skin treatments

If you find staff devoting time and resources to these items, you are well within proper boundaries to skill a resident.

Section 30.2.4: Questionable situations

Section 30.2.4 briefly addresses some "questionable situations."

There must be specific evidence that daily skilled nursing or skilled rehabilitation services are required and received if:

- *The primary service needed is oral medication; or*

- *The patient is capable of independent ambulation, dressing, feeding, and hygiene.*

Although this section may seem brief, note the last statement: whether the patient "is capable of independent ambulation, dressing, feeding, and hygiene." This will be important when determining whether a patient is skillable when completing the MDS, and especially when you consider the impact that these items have on the portion of the resource utilization group (RUG) score pertaining to activities of daily living. Although the MDS does not determine skilled care needs, it must support the need for skilled care.

Section 30.3: Direct skilled nursing services to patients

Skilling under this section tends to be easier, as the services are tangible rather than cognitive. Section 30.3 provides some examples of what is considered to be "skilled nursing":

- Intravenous or intramuscular injections and intravenous feeding.

- Enteral feeding that composes at least 26% of daily calorie requirements and provides at least 501 mL of fluid per day.

- Nasopharyngeal and tracheotomy aspiration.

- Insertion, sterile irrigation, and replacement of suprapubic catheters.

- Application of dressings involving prescription medications and aseptic techniques.

- Treatment of decubitus ulcers of a severity rated at Stage 3 or worse, or of a widespread skin disorder.

- Heat treatments that have been specifically ordered by a physician as part of active treatment and that require observation by skilled nursing personnel to adequately evaluate the resident's progress.

- Rehabilitation nursing procedures, including the related teaching and adaptive aspects of nursing that are part of active treatment and require the presence of skilled nursing personnel (e.g., the institution and supervision of bowel and bladder training programs).

- Initial phases of a regimen involving administration of medical gases, such as bronchodilator therapy.

- Care of a colostomy during the early postoperative period in the presence of associated complications. The need for skilled nursing care during this period must be justified and documented in the resident's medical record.

It is crucial to keep in mind that the services previously identified must take place in accordance with Section 30.2, which mandates the direct care or general supervision of a licensed professional.

Section 30.4.1.1: Direct skilled rehabilitation services to patients

Section 30.4.1.1 dictates the following related to skilled rehabilitation services to SNF residents under Medicare:

- *The services must be directly and specifically related to an active written treatment plan that is based upon an initial evaluation performed by a qualified physical therapist after admission to the SNF and prior to the start of physical therapy services in the SNF that is approved by the physician after any needed consultation with the qualified physical therapist. In those cases where a beneficiary is discharged during the SNF stay and later readmitted, an initial evaluation must be performed upon readmission to the SNF, prior to the start of physical therapy services in the SNF.*

- *The services must be of a level of complexity and sophistication, or the condition of the patient must be of a nature that requires the judgment, knowledge, and skills of a qualified physical therapist;*

- *The services must be provided with the expectation, based on the assessment made by the physician of the patient's restoration potential, that the condition of the patient will improve materially in a reasonable and generally predictable period of time, or the services must be necessary for the establishment of a safe and effective maintenance program;*

- *The services must be considered under accepted standards of medical practice to be specific and effective treatment for the patient's condition; and*

- *The services must be reasonable and necessary for the treatment of the patient's condition; this includes the requirement that the amount, frequency, and duration of the services must be reasonable.*

Keep in mind that the treatments rendered must require the services of a qualified therapy professional. There are several different services that a resident might require that can be provided by a nonlicensed individual or support staff member; it is imperative to identify that the skilled therapy services require the skills of a licensed professional. These nonskilled services might involve general exercise to promote overall fitness and flexibility and activities to provider diversion or general motivation.

This section of the manual also offers examples, such as residents who require therapy services to restore functions lost as a result of muscle atrophy after surgery or illness, and a resident who had a double amputation surgery. The resident needed therapy to help with transfers, bed mobility, and wheelchair mobility.

As you examine the manual for examples of reasonable and necessary SLP and OT, you will see that it refers the reader to Chapter 1, "Inpatient Hospital Services" of the *Medicare Benefit Policy Manual*. Therefore, as you read Chapter 1 of the *Medicare Benefit Policy Manual*, note that the emphasis and guidelines are the same for PT, OT, and SLP as for PT or therapy in general, as discussed earlier when we talked about Section 30.4.1.1. Ultimately, you have at least two references or sources for therapy: Section 30.4.1.1 and Chapter 1 of the *Medicare Benefit Policy Manual*.

Section 30.4.1.2 identifies the following as some of the more common skilled physical therapy modalities and procedures related to skilled services in a SNF:

- **Assessment**—The skills of a physical therapist are required for the ongoing assessment of a patient's rehabilitation needs and potential.

- **Therapeutic exercise**—Therapeutic exercise, which must be performed by or under the supervision of the qualified physical therapist, due to either the type of exercise employed or the condition of the patient.

- **Gait training**—Gait evaluation and training furnished to a patient whose agility to walk has been impaired by neurological, muscular, or skeletal abnormality often require the skills of a qualified physical therapist.

- **Range of motion**—Such exercises constitute skilled physical therapy only if they are part of an active treatment for a specific disease state that has resulted in the loss or restriction of mobility. Only the qualified therapist may perform such tests.

- **Maintenance therapy**—The repetitive services required to maintain function sometimes involve the use of complex and sophisticated therapy procedures, and, consequently, the judgment and skills of a physical therapist might be required for the safe and effective rendition of such services.

- **Ultrasound, shortwave, and microwave diathermy**

- **Hot packs, infrared treatments, paraffin baths, and whirlpool baths**—Such treatments of this type do not ordinarily require the skills of a qualified therapist; however, the skills, knowledge, and judgment of a qualified therapist might be required in the rendering of such treatments depending on the specific resident situation.

Information related to speech language pathology and occupational therapy can be found in Chapter 1 "Inpatient Hospital Services" of the *Medicare Benefit Policy Manual*.

We have made a thorough review of what Medicare considers to be "skilled" services in a SNF under Medicare Part A. Now, let us review what services are not considered "skilled" in nature and are often referred to as nonskilled, intermediate, or custodial care services in the industry.

Section 30.5: Nonskilled supportive or personal care services

This section starts out with the following disclaimer, if you will: *"The following services are not skilled services unless rendered under circumstances detailed in Section 30.2."* We will revisit this statement after we review the services listed in this section as being nonskilled, supportive, or personal care services. Such services listed in this section include the following:

- *Administration of routine oral medications, eye drops, and ointments. The fact that residents cannot be relied upon to take such medications themselves or that state law requires all medications to be dispensed by a nurse to institutional patients would not change this service to a skilled service.*

- *General maintenance care of colostomy and ileostomy.*

- *Routine services to maintain satisfactory functioning of indwelling bladder catheters, including emptying and cleaning containers and clamping the tubing.*

- *Changes of dressings for uninfected postoperative or chronic conditions.*

- *Prophylactic and palliative skin care, including bathing and application of creams or treatment of minor skin problems.*

- *Routine care of the incontinent resident, including use of diapers and protective sheets.*

- *General maintenance care in connection with a plaster cast. Skilled supervision or observation may be required where the resident has a preexisting skin or circulatory condition or requires adjustment of traction.*

- *Routine care in connection with braces and similar devices.*

- *Use of heat as a palliative and comfort measure, such as via whirlpool or steam pack.*

- *Routine administration of medical gases after a regimen of therapy has been established (i.e., administration of medical gases after the patient has been taught how to institute therapy).*

- *Assistance in dressing, eating, and toileting.*

- *Periodic turning and positioning in bed.*

- *General supervision of exercises that have been taught to the resident and the performance of repetitious exercises that do not require skilled rehabilitation personnel for their performance. This includes the actual administration of maintenance programs in which the performances of repetitive exercises that may be required to maintain function do not necessitate the involvement and services of skilled rehabilitation personnel. It also includes the carrying out of repetitive exercises to improve gait or maintain strength or endurance, passive exercises not related to a specific loss of function to maintain range of motion in paralyzed extremities, and assistive walking. (See the* Medicare Benefit Policy Manual, *Chapter 1, "Inpatient Hospital Services.")*

Now, back to the disclaimer: "The following services are not skilled services unless rendered under circumstances detailed in Section 30.2." This is extremely important. In other words, if any of the services listed within Section 30.5 take place without the general supervision or direct care of a licensed professional, they cannot be considered skillable services.

However, if services listed in Section 30.5 take place under the general supervision or direct care of a licensed professional, these items can be considered skilled. Just as we have reviewed in earlier chapters, that diagnosis alone cannot qualify a resident for Medicare Part A services in a SNF; the same principles apply in this instance. Services themselves cannot determine the skilled status of a resident; rather, we have to review the resident's total plan of care and maintenance and who is providing the services in the bigger picture, and not just focus on the types of services being rendered.

We have now thoroughly defined the requirements for skilled services in the SNF. All of these services from the manual are listed for a reason. First, in case you decide to never crack open the CMS manuals, you can read about these services right here; second, and more importantly, this will get your attention with regard to the simplicity of what might be involved in skilled care. It will become even clearer as we tie this information to the MDS requirements.

Next, we need to review the requirement that the services be ordered by a physician and what requirements, time frames, and parameters are required with what is referred to as a physician certification and recertification.

Section 40: Physician Certification and Recertification of Extended Care Services

A physician must certify or recertify on a regular basis that a resident still needs particular treatments or care. However, a NP or clinical nurse specialist (CNS) may also certify and recertify for these purposes as well. The certification must clearly indicate that posthospital extended care services were required to be given on an inpatient basis because of the individual's need for skilled care on a continuing basis for any of the conditions for which he or she was receiving inpatient hospital services. There is no specific procedure or form required by CMS to meet this requirement. This section of the manual specifically states: "There is no requirement for a specific procedure or form as long as the approach adopted by the facility permits verification that the certification and recertification requirement is met."

Certification or recertification statements may be entered on or included in forms, notes, or other records that a physician, NP, or CNS normally signs in caring for a patient, or may be included on a separate form. Except as otherwise specified, each certification and recertification is to be signed by a physician, NP, or CNS.

This allows SNFs the autonomy to adopt a procedure that best fits individual needs or situations. However, many SNFs will adopt a form to use for this purpose to ease the process of verification of the physician certification prior to billing.

Who may sign the certification or recertification for extended care services

According to Section 40.1:

> *A certification or recertification statement must be signed by the attending physician or a physician on the staff of the skilled nursing facility who has knowledge of the case, or by a nurse practitioner (NP) or clinical nurse specialist (CNS) who does not have a direct or indirect employment relationship with the facility, but who is working in collaboration with the physician.*

Often a SNF may ask a medical director to sign if the attending physician is unavailable during the time when the recertification is required, for instance. In such cases, as long as the medical director has knowledge of the case and is willing to sign such a practice is acceptable based on this section of the regulation.

The initial certification must be obtained at the time of admission or as soon thereafter as is reasonable and practicable, according to the manual. Many facilities adopt a rule of within 72 hours of admission, which has been acceptable to CMS. CMS also indicates that a routine admission order by a physician, NP, or CNS does not meet the qualification for this requirement. "There must be a separate signed statement indicating that the patient will require on a daily basis SNF covered care."

We will refer to Section 40 of Chapter 4 of Publication 100-01, *Medicare General Information, Eligibility and Entitlement,* for the following additional information:

- Certification and recertification language

- Timing of recertifications

- Impact of failure to obtain a certification or recertification

Certification and recertification language

Per Section 40.2 of this publication:

> The **certification** *must clearly indicate that posthospital extended care services were required to be given on an inpatient basis because of the individual's need for skilled care on a continuing basis for any of the conditions for which he/she was receiving inpatient hospital services, including services of an emergency hospital.*

Additionally, this same section indicates that:

> The **recertification** *statement must contain an adequate written record of the reasons for the continued need for extended care services, the estimated period of time required for the patient to remain in the facility, and any plans, where appropriate, for home care. The recertification statement made by the physician does not have to include this entire statement if, for example, all of the required information is in fact included in progress notes.*

If the physician, NP, or CNS does not include the referenced statement related to continued need for extended care services, he or she must reference the section of the medical record that contains that information. The manual specifically states that, "A statement reciting only that continued extended care services are medically necessary is not, in and of itself, sufficient." In addition, the physician, NP, or CNS must also document on recertifications any additional issues that have arose since admission from the hospital that contribute to the continued need for skilled services in the SNF.

Timing of recertifications

As noted, the initial certification has to occur at the time of admission or soon thereafter. The initial recertification must be made no later than the 14th day of inpatient skilled services. However, CMS allows the physician to sign an initial certification and one more recertification at the same time. Additional recertifications are required, at a minimum, every 30 days thereafter. SNFs have the ability to recertify in shorter intervals, as desired, but the maximum length of a period between recertifications is 30 days.

One common pitfall is the assumption that this statement indicates that recertifications are required by days 14, 44, and 74 of the stay in all cases. Let us review the following example:

- A resident is admitted on October 1 and the initial certification and recertification are both signed on day three of the stay. Subsequent recertifications are required every 30 days. In this instance, then, the next recertification would be required by November 1, which is 30 days from the initial recertification signed on October 3, but only day 32 of the resident's stay. If the SNF assumed that the recertification was due on day 44, the window would have been missed and there would be a gap in the recertification and services would not be billable to the program.

It is important to make sure staff understand that the timing of the recertifications is not set in stone; rather, it is dependent on when the initial recertification and subsequent recertifications are actually completed and signed.

Impact of failure to obtain a certification or recertification

As we noted at the beginning of this chapter, one of the four requirements for covering and billing for skilled services in the SNF is that a physician, NP, or CNS has certified the need for services in the SNF. Therefore, failure to obtain such certification would preclude the SNF from billing the services to Medicare for reimbursement. There is some language in Section 40.5 of the manual that discusses delays in certifications or recertifications.

> *[D]elayed certifications and recertifications will be honored where, for example, there has been an isolated oversight or lapse. In addition to complying with the content requirements, delayed certifications and recertifications must include an explanation for the delay and any medical or other evidence which the skilled nursing facility considers relevant for purposes of explaining the delay. The facility will determine the format of delayed certification and recertification statements, and the method by which they are obtained. A delayed certification and recertification may appear in one statement; separate signed statements for each certification and recertification would not be required as they would if timely certification and recertification had been made.*

Although SNFs are not required to transmit the physician certification and recertification information to CMS to validate coverage, these documents will be requested upon any type of medical review to validate that the requirements have been met. It is the expectation of CMS that SNFs certify the presence and completeness of physician certifications and recertifications prior to submitting a claim for reimbursement for Medicare Part A SNF services.

After all that, you might be asking yourself, "How can I possibly know all of the needs of my resident before they are admitted to even know if they qualify for skilled services in my SNF?" So glad you asked ... let us review the administrative presumption criteria next.

Section 30.1: Administrative presumption (exception to skilled coverage rule for a specified time period)

Section 30.1 features a relatively brief explanation of how residents are preliminarily assessed by the MDS and are classified into RUG categories. Under the SNF prospective payment system (PPS), beneficiaries who are admitted (or readmitted) directly to a SNF after a qualifying hospital stay are considered to meet the level-of-care requirements of 42 CFR 409.31 automatically. The time frame for this exception is up to and including the assessment reference date for the five-day or return/readmission Medicare assessment. Note again, there is no set time frame; you do not automatically get three days, five days, eight days, etc. It is up to the point when you determine that services are truly not skilled in nature that you must discontinue. The presumption gives you time to review, assess, and evaluate, but it does not provide for a set period of time to accomplish those processes. Presumption is only valid when the beneficiary is correctly assigned to one of the RUG payment categories designated as representing the required level of care (i.e., the top 52 RUG categories from extensive plus rehab to clinically complex). This section requires an accurately completed MDS form, and if the patient classifies below the top 52 payment categories (see Figure 3.1), clinical documentation is needed to support the daily skilled need.

FIGURE
3.1

Top 52 RUG-IV categories

Rehabilitation plus extensive services	RUX, RUL, RVX, RVL, RHX, RHL, RMX, RML, RLX
Rehabilitation	RUA, RUB, RUC, RVA, RVB, RVC, RHA, RHB, RHC, RMA, RMB, RMC, RLA, RLB
Extensive services	ES3, ES2, ES1
Special care high	HE2, HE1, HD2, HD1, HC2, HC1, HB2, HB1
Special care low	LE2, LE1, LD2, LD1, LC2, LC1, LB2, LB1
Clinically complex	CE2, CE1, CD2, CD1, CC2, CC1, CB2, CB1, CA2, CA1

It is important to note, as indicated in Section 30.1, that:

A beneficiary who groups into other than one of the RUGs designated as representing the required level of care on the 5-day assessment prescribed in 42 CFR 413.343(b) is not automatically classified as meeting or not meeting the SNF level of care definition. Instead, the beneficiary must receive an individual level of care determination using existing administrative criteria and procedures.

Another important criteria to note is that administrative presumption can only apply with direct admits to the SNF from a qualifying hospital stay. If a resident discharges to home and then comes to the SNF for admission (within the 30-day window) administrative presumption is not valid in that instance. In addition, administrative presumption also does not apply in a SNF-to-SNF transfer situation.

There are still a few more areas we have not reviewed in detail as of yet. We understand that skilled services are required and what administrative presumption is, but what about the following:

- The patient requires these skilled services on a daily basis

- As a practical matter, considering economy and efficiency, the daily skilled services can be provided only on an inpatient basis in a SNF

Well, we have tackled the two most difficult of the four criteria mentioned in the beginning of this chapter, with only two left, so we are half-way there. Actually, the last two criteria require less explanation.

Section 30.6: Daily skilled services defined

Section 30.6 provides some information for you to memorize and to which you must adhere. For instance, skilled nursing services or skilled rehabilitation services must be needed on a daily basis. To meet the "daily" need as a rehab resident, the resident must receive therapy five days per week.

CMS elaborates that this requirement is not to be interpreted so strictly that it would not be met because of an isolated break or two in therapy within a seven-day period. Also, do not forget that in order to meet a rehab low RUG category, only three days of licensed therapy per week must be provided in conjunction with restorative therapy for six days per week.

Section 30.7: Services provided on an inpatient basis as a practical matter

Section 30.7 brings up an issue that we do not encounter too often: whether a resident can receive care from an alternative source.

> As a "practical matter," daily skilled services can be provided only in a SNF if they are not available on an outpatient basis in the area in which the individual resides or transportation to the closest facility would be:
>
> - An excessive physical hardship;
>
> - Less economical; or
>
> - Less efficient or effective than an inpatient institutional setting.
>
> The availability of capable and willing family or the feasibility of obtaining other assistance for the patient at home should be considered. Even though needed daily skilled services might be available on an outpatient or home care basis, as a practical matter, the care can be furnished only in the SNF if home care would be ineffective because the patient would have insufficient assistance at home to reside there safely.

Most of the time, when residents come to a SNF, they are there because all other resources have been considered and rejected. However, sometimes residents can get the level of care they need from home health or from an outpatient therapy clinic. Keep in mind that many of the care alternatives have been explored by the physician, family, and hospital discharge planner before the facility has even considered skilling a patient.

Ultimately, everyone involved (including the facility) must agree that the care can be provided only on an inpatient basis.

The question of daily skilled services and the practical matter criteria is often questioned more during the holiday season with the question of "Can a resident go home for the holidays?" A common misconception is that a Medicare Part A resident's absence from the facility for any period of time jeopardizes the resident's coverage under the program. However, that is not the case.

To answer this question, we need to review several different areas of the regulation. First of all, can the resident safely be absent from the facility for the period of time? The SNF staff needs to review the resident's condition and evaluate what is involved in the individual resident's care plan that might impact the ability to be gone for any period of time. In addition, is there an individual or family member who is capable of providing any of those care needs during the absence, and what will be required to teach that individual or family member to care for the resident during the temporary absence? Section 30.7.3 of Chapter 8 of the manual clearly states:

> *Decisions in these cases should be based on information reflecting the care needed and received by the patient while in the SNF and on the arrangements needed for the provision, if any, of this care during any absences.*

A resident who is near the end of their Part A stay for a knee replacement, with no other complications, who was previously living independently, may very well be a good candidate for an absence from the SNF for a special occasion.

However, the following resident may not be a good candidate for a leave of absence due to the myriad of issues and concerns and the difficulty to be able to teach a friend or family member to provide the necessary care during the leave.

Mrs. T, an 83-year-old female was admitted to the facility one week ago following a left hip fracture with open reduction, internal fixation (ORIF). She had fallen at home after tripping on a throw rug in her kitchen. She has had increasing dysphagia for the past four months, noticing coughing at intervals after drinking water and feeling like food is going down the wrong way. She suffers from orthostatic hypotension when changing positions from sitting to standing and experiences shortness of breath with minimal activity, being observed to have an increased respiratory rate and audible respirations. She is continent of bowel and bladder. She currently has no evident pressure ulcers, but her tissue tolerance identifies she needs repositioning every one to one and a half hours.

The second item that needs to be reviewed is whether that absence will jeopardize the resident's ability to meet that "practical matter" criteria discussed earlier in this chapter. We will refer to Section 30.7.3 of the manual again:

While most beneficiaries requiring a SNF level of care find that they are unable to leave the facility, the fact that a patient is granted an outside pass or short leave of absence for the purpose of attending a special religious service, holiday meal, family occasion, going on a car ride, or for a trial visit home, is not, by itself evidence that the individual no longer needs to be in a SNF for the receipt of required skilled care.

However, the manual does go a step further in reminding SNFs that if the absences from the SNF are frequent or for prolonged periods of time, it is possible that their need for SNF placement and that "practical matter" criteria could come into question.

So we can be comfortable encouraging residents to go home for special occasions if SNF staff feel that residents can safely be away from the SNF and their family can be instructed to meet their care needs; and if the absences are not frequent in nature, or for prolonged periods of time. Each resident and leave of absence has to be reviewed independently and as it occurs to determine whether it is feasible under the two criteria identified. To have a standing policy or to communicate to a Medicare Part A resident that leaving the facility for a short absence will jeopardize their coverage is not appropriate, each situation has to be evaluated on a case-by-case basis.

It is important to also address the situation of charging the resident privately for a bed hold during a temporary absence as well, as this issue is surrounded by much confusion. In the *Medicare Claims*

Processing Manual, Chapter 1, Section 30.1.1.1, it states that a SNF is permitted to charge a beneficiary for a bed hold during a temporary absence from the SNF. In addition, under §1819(c)(1)(B)(iii) of the Social Security Act and 42 CFR 483.10 (b)(5) through (6):

> [T]he facility must inform residents in advance of their option to make bed-hold payments, as well as the amount of the facility's charge. For these optional payments, the facility should make clear that the resident must affirmatively elect to make them prior to being billed. A facility cannot simply deem a resident to have opted to make such payments and then automatically bill for them upon the resident's departure from the facility.

That said, it is also important to recognize that from a federal perspective a SNF has no obligation to hold a resident's bed during temporary absences from the SNF; however, each state may have specific guidance related to this process. Additionally, most state medical assistance programs also have specific requirements for bed holds for dual eligible residents that should also be reviewed if the SNF is a provider in their state medical assistance program.

Take a Deep Breath

Although Chapter 8 of Publication 100-02 contains several other sections, they really do not help you to understand how to increase your skilled census of residents. However, as we look back at the prior text, we have covered a lot of ground. As we move into Chapter 4, we will begin taking a more in-depth look at skilled service provision by reviewing the MDS process in detail.

MDS 3.0—Assessments, Selection, and Sections ... Oh My!

The minimum data set (MDS) does not determine skilled need. Actual determination of skilled need must be based on the regulatory criteria discussed in the earlier chapters of this book. However, just as a barometer uses atmospheric pressure to predict and confirm changing weather conditions, humidity, and storms, the MDS is a predictive and confirming measure.

The MDS provides support for daily skilled need, alerts the staff to potential changes in the clinical condition of a patient, and establishes the link to receive payment for providing skilled care. From delivery of therapy minutes to cognitive loss to functional level, the MDS assessment and the related documentation supply evidence of care, care delivery, evaluation of risk factors, improvements, and declines. It measures or assesses Medicare patients on a more frequent basis than non-Medicare residents are assessed. This allows you to capture the subtle changes to clinical conditions that should prompt reassessment of a resident's daily skilled need.

Mastering many resources is required to successfully navigate any component of the Medicare spectrum, including skilled care. The MDS is fundamental to the process and represents an interdisciplinary view of the patient. The MDS is one component of the resident assessment instrument (RAI) process and a critical component in the delivery of skilled care.

Brief History of MDS 3.0

Before we begin an in-depth look at the MDS and all of the processes involved, we should briefly review the history of the MDS 3.0, which was implemented on October 1, 2010, and represented the most significant change to the MDS and skilled nursing facility (SNF) reimbursement since 1998. According to the Centers for Medicare & Medicaid Services (CMS) website:

> The MDS is a powerful tool for implementing standardized assessment and for facilitating care manage-
> ment in nursing homes (NHs) and non-critical access hospital swing beds (SBs). Its content has

implications for residents, families, providers, researchers, and policymakers, all of whom have expressed concerns about the reliability, validity, and relevance of MDS 2.0. Some argue that because MDS 2.0 fails to include items that rely on direct resident interview, it fails to obtain critical information and effectively disenfranchises many residents from the assessment process. In addition, many users and government agencies have expressed concerns about MDS 2.0 data quality and validity. Other stakeholders contend that items used in other care settings should be included to improve communication across providers.

MDS 3.0 has been designed to improve the reliability, accuracy, and usefulness of the MDS, to include the resident in the assessment process, and to use standard protocols used in other settings. These improvements have profound implications for NH [nursing home] and SB [swing bed] care and public policy. Enhanced accuracy supports the primary legislative intent that MDS be a tool to improve clinical assessment and supports the credibility of programs that rely on MDS.

In creating the new assessment tool, CMS rolled out a national initiative to create MDS 3.0. According to the final report issued by Rand Health, who published the "Development and Validation of a Revised Nursing Home Assessment Tool: MDS 3.0", the purpose of the study was to "[i]mprove the clinical relevance and accuracy of MDS assessments, increase the voice of residents in assessments, improve user satisfaction, and increase the efficiency of reports."

The major findings, published by that same report, were as follows:

- **Accuracy:** MDS 3.0 items showed either excellent or very good reliability even when comparing research nurse to facility–nurse assessments. For items that were validated against criterion measures, the MDS 3.0 performed better than MDS 2.0.

- **Resident voice:** MDS 3.0 successfully included resident voice. The majority of residents were able to complete interview sections. Staff members reported that items provided useful clinical insights; analyses showed improved validity for cognitive and mood items.

- **Clinical relevance:** Nurses who used MDS 3.0 reported that the revisions were more clinically relevant and useful than MDS 2.0; items used in other clinical settings showed either excellent or very good reliability with low rates of missing responses when tested in MDS 3.0.

- **Efficiency:** MDS 3.0 improved assessments while decreasing the time to complete them. The average time for completing the MDS 3.0 was 45% less than the average time for MDS 2.0, based on the same sample.

- **Crosswalk:** Although MDS 3.0 improved detection of clinical problems, items could be mapped to MDS 2.0 payment cells in a manner that avoided significant shifts in payment.

Now that we have a brief understanding of the "why" related to the MDS 3.0, let us begin reviewing the "how."

Types of MDS Assessments

According to *42 CFR §483.20*, the SNF must conduct initial and periodic assessments to assess a resident's functional capacity. The *RAI User's Manual* (published by CMS for the MDS 3.0) identifies the following requirements for potential long-term care resident assessments:

- All residents of Medicare SNFs or Medicaid (Title 19) nursing facilities

- Hospice residents

- Short-term or respite residents

Assessments are grouped into two basic categories:

1. Medicare-required prospective payment system (PPS) assessments

2. Omnibus Budget Reconciliation Act of 1987 (OBRA)–required assessments

Medicare-required PPS assessments are specific to residents in a Medicare Part A SNF stay and provide information relevant to SNF reimbursement under resource utilization group (RUG)-IV PPS. OBRA-required assessments are federally mandated and are required to be performed on all residents in a nursing home that is certified by either Medicare (Title 18) or Medicaid (Title 19). Depending on timing and circumstance, there is the option to combine these assessments into one assessment.

Figure 4.1 identifies the different types of assessments under both Medicare PPS and OBRA. Figure 4.2 identifies all of the different stand-alone and combinations of the assessments possible under both requirements. It is stressed though, that when an assessment is combined, the more stringent requirements of their Medicare or OBRA must be applied.

FIGURE *4.1*	Types of assessments—Medicare- and OBRA-required

Medicare-required PPS Assessments
5 day
14 day
30 day
60 day
90 day
Readmission/Return
Significant Changes in Status Assessment (SCSA)
Significant Correction to Prior Assessment (SCPA)
Swing Bed Clinical Change (CCA)
Start of Therapy (SOT) Other Medicare Required Assessment (OMRA)
End of Therapy (EOT) OMRA
Both SOT and EOT OMRA
OBRA-required Assessments
Entry Record
Admission (comprehensive)
Quarterly
Annual (comprehensive)
Significant Changes in Status Assessment (SCSA) (comprehensive)
Significant Correction to Prior Assessment (SCPA) (comprehensive)
Significant Change in Quarterly Assessment (SCQA)
Discharge – Return not anticipated
Discharge – Return anticipated
Death in Facility

FIGURE
4.2

MDS 3.0 HIPPS modifiers

Code	Narrative Description
00	Default
01	Unscheduled PPS/unscheduled (OBRA)
02	Unscheduled PPS/SOT OMRA
03	Unscheduled PPS/unscheduled SOT/OMRA + unscheduled OBRA
04	Unscheduled PPS/EOT OMRA whether or not combined with unscheduled OBRA
05	Unscheduled PPS/SOT OMRA + EOT OMRA
06	Unscheduled PPS/SOT OMRA + EOT OMRA + unscheduled OBRA
07	Unscheduled PPS Medicare SSA
10	PPS 5-day or readmission return
11	PPS 5-day or readmission return/unscheduled OBRA
12	PPS 5-day or readmission return/SOT OMRA
13	PPS 5-day or readmission return/SOT OMRA + unscheduled OBRA
14	PPS 5-day or readmission return/EOT OMRA whether or not combined with unscheduled OBRA
15	PPS 5-day or readmission return/SOT OMRA + EOT OMRA
16	PPS 5-day or readmission return/SOT OMRA + EOT OMRA + unscheduled OBRA
17	PPS 5-day or readmission return/Medicare SSA
20	PPS 14-day
21	PPS 14-day/unscheduled OBRA
22	PPS 14-day/SOT OMRA
23	PPS 14-day/SOT OMRA + unscheduled OBRA
24	PPS 14-day/EOT OMRA whether or not combined with unscheduled OBRA
25	PPS 14-day/SOT OMRA + EOT OMRA
26	PPS 14-day/SOT OMRA + EOT OMRA + unscheduled OBRA
27	PPS 14-day/Medicare SSA
30	PPS 30-day
31	PPS 30-day/unscheduled OBRA

FIGURE
4.2

MDS 3.0 HIPPS modifiers (cont.)

Code	Narrative Description
32	PPS 30-day/SOT OMRA
33	PPS 30-day/SOT OMRA + unscheduled ORA
34	PPS 30-day EOT OMRA whether or not combined with unscheduled OBRA
35	PPS 30-day/SOT OMRA + EOT OMRA
36	PPS 30-day/SOT OMRA + EOT OMRA + unscheduled OBRA
37	PPS 30-day/Medicare SSA
40	PPS 60-day
41	PPS 60-day/unscheduled OBRA
42	PPS 60-day/SOT OMRA
43	PPS 60-day/SOT + unscheduled OBRA
44	PPS 60-day/EOT OMRA whether or not combined with unscheduled OBRA
45	PPS 60-day/SOT OMRA + EOT OMRA
46	PPS 60-day/SOT OMRA + EOT OMRA + unscheduled OBRA
47	PPS 60-day/Medicare SSA
50	PPS 90–day
51	PPS 90-day/either an unscheduled OBRA
52	PPS 90-day/SOT OMRA
53	PPS 90-day/SOT + unscheduled OBRA
54	PPS 90-day/EOT OMRA whether or not combined with unscheduled OBRA
55	PPS 90-day/SOT OMRA + EOT OMRA
56	PPS 90-day/SOT OMRA + EOT OMRA + unscheduled OBRA
57	PPS 90-day/ Medicare SSA
60	OBRA used for PPS
61	OBRA used for PPS unscheduled OBRA
62	OBRA used for PPS/SOT OMRA
63	OBRA used for PPS/SOT OMRA combined with an unscheduled OBRA

FIGURE
4.2

MDS 3.0 HIPPS modifiers (cont.)

Code	Narrative Description
64	OBRA used for PPS PPS/EOT OMRA whether or not combined with unscheduled OBRA
65	OBRA used for PPS/SOT OMRA + EOT OMRA
66	OBRA used for PPS/SOT OMRA + EOT OMRA + unscheduled OBRA
67	OBRA used for PPS/Medicare SSA
Acronyms	
OBRA	Scheduled assessment (14 days of adm., Q = ≤ 92 days, annual = ≤ 366 days
OMRA	Other Medicare-related assessment
SOT	Start of therapy (OPTIONAL)
EOT	End of therapy
SSA	Short stay assessment
Entry	Must always have one (on admission or readmission)
Discharge	Must always have one (except for leave of absence [LOA])

Listed as follows is a brief explanation from the *RAI User's Manual* on the different types of assessments.

Admission assessment

The admission assessment is a comprehensive assessment for a new resident and, under some circumstances, a returning resident that must be completed by the end of day 14, counting the date of admission to the nursing home as day one if any of the following are met:

- This is the resident's first time in this facility

- The resident had been in this facility previously and was discharged prior to completion of the OBRA admission assessment

- The resident has been admitted to this facility and was discharged with a return not anticipated

- The resident has been admitted to this facility and was discharged with a return anticipated and did not return within 30 days of discharge

Quarterly assessment

The quarterly assessment is an OBRA noncomprehensive assessment for a resident that must be completed at least every 92 days following the previous OBRA assessment of any type. It is used to track a resident's status between comprehensive assessments to ensure that any critical indicators of gradual change in a resident's status are monitored. As such, not all MDS items appear on the quarterly assessment. The assessment reference date (ARD) (Item A2300) must not be more than 92 days after the ARD of the most recent OBRA assessment of any type.

Annual assessment

The annual assessment is a comprehensive assessment for a resident that must be completed on an annual basis (at least every 366 days) unless a significant change in status assessment (SCSA) or a significant correction to prior comprehensive assessment (SCPA) has been completed since the most recent comprehensive assessment was completed. Its completion dates (MDS/care area assessments [CAA]/care plan) depend on the most recent comprehensive and past assessments' ARDs and completion dates.

Significant change in status assessment (SCSA)

The SCSA is a comprehensive assessment for a resident that must be completed when the interdisciplinary team (IDT) has determined that a resident meets the significant change guidelines for either improvement or decline. It can be performed at any time after the completion of an admission assessment, and its completion dates (MDS/CAA(s)/care plan) depend on the date that the IDT's determination was made that the resident had a significant change.

Significant correction to prior comprehensive assessment (SCPA)

The SCPA is a comprehensive assessment for an existing resident that must be completed when the IDT determines that a resident's prior comprehensive assessment contains a significant error. It can be performed at any time after the completion of an admission assessment, and its ARD and completion dates

(MDS/CAA(s)/care plan) depend on the date the determination was made that a significant error existed in a comprehensive assessment.

Significant correction to prior quarterly assessment (SCQA)

The SCQA is an OBRA noncomprehensive assessment for a resident that must be completed when the IDT determines that a resident's prior quarterly assessment contains a significant error. It can be performed at any time after the completion of a quarterly assessment, and the ARD (Item A2300) and completion dates (Item Z0500B) depend on the date the determination was made that there is a significant error in a previous quarterly assessment.

Start of therapy (SOT) Other Medicare-Required Assessment (OMRA)

The SOT OMRA is optional and completed only to classify a resident into a RUG-IV Rehabilitation Plus Extensive Services group or Rehabilitation group. If the RUG-IV classification is not a Rehabilitation Plus Extensive Services or a Rehabilitation (therapy) group, the assessment will not be accepted by CMS and cannot be used for Medicare billing. It is also completed only if the resident is not already classified into a RUG-IV Rehabilitation Plus Extensive Services or Rehabilitation group.

End of therapy (EOT) OMRA

The EOT OMRA is required when a resident is classified in a RUG-IV Rehabilitation Plus Extensive Services or Rehabilitation group and continues to need Part A SNF-level services after the discontinuation of all rehabilitation therapies.

Medicare short-stay assessment

To be considered a Medicare short-stay assessment and use the special RUG-IV short-stay rehabilitation therapy classification, the assessment must be a SOT OMRA, the resident must have been discharged from Part A on or before day eight of the Part A stay, and the resident must have completed only one to four days of therapy, with therapy having started during the last four days of the Part A stay. To be considered a Medicare short-stay assessment and use the special RUG-IV short-stay rehabilitation therapy classification, there are eight specific criteria that have to be met. SNF staff are encouraged to refer to Chapter 6 of the *RAI User's Manual* for additional information on coding this assessment.

FIGURE 4.3	Minimum required item set by assessment type for skilled nursing facilities		

	Comprehensive Item Set	Quarterly/PPS* Item Sets	Other Required Assessments/Tracking Item Sets for Skilled Nursing Facilities
Stand-alone Assessment Types	• OBRA admission • Annual • Significant change in status (SCSA) • Significant correction to prior comprehensive (SCPA)	• Quarterly • Significant correction to prior quarterly • PPS 5-day (5-day) • PPS 14-day (14-day) • PPS 30-day (30-day) • PPS 60-day (60-day) • PPS 90-day (90-day) • PPS readmission/return	• Entry tracking record • Discharge assessments • Death in facility tracking record • Start of therapy OMRA • Start of therapy OMRA and discharge • OMRA • OMRA and discharge
Combined Assessment Types	• OBRA admission and 5-day • OBRA admission and 14-Day • OBRA admission and any OMRA • Annual and any Medicare-required • Annual and any OMRA • SCSA and any Medicare-required • SCSA and any OMRA • SCPA and any Medicare-required • SCPA and any OMRA • Any OBRA comprehensive and any discharge	• Quarterly and any Medicare-scheduled • Quarterly and any OMRA • Significant correction to prior quarterly and any Medicare-required • Significant correction to prior quarterly and any OMRA • Any discharge and any Medicare-required • Quarterly and any discharge • Significant correction to prior quarterly and any discharge • Any Medicare-required and any discharge	N/A

* Provider must check with state agency to determine if the state requires additional items to be completed for the required OBRA quarterly and PPS assessments.

Source: The RAI User's Manual.

What Makes an Assessment Comprehensive?

A comprehensive assessment requires that the MDS process, the CAA process, and care plan be completed. Comprehensive assessments are required as follows:

- Upon admission

- On an annual basis

- Upon significant change in status

- Upon significant correction of a prior comprehensive assessment

---

CAA

The review of one or more of the 20 conditions, symptoms, and other areas of concern that are commonly identified or suggested by MDS findings. Care areas are triggered by responses on the MDS item set. There is an entire appendix of the *RAI User's Manual* dedicated to CAA resources in Appendix C. We will not be reviewing this process in detail in this book as it does not relate to the determination of skilled services, but rather additional assessments required that are based on the 20 care area triggers derived from information entered into the MDS.

The Assessment Schedule

There are four important components to understanding the timing involved in the Medicare/OBRA assessment schedule.

- ARD

- Look-back period

- Completion date

- Transmission date

ARD

The ARD refers to the last day of the look-back period through which assessment information can be gathered. Upon admission of a resident, the registered nurse assessment coordinator (RNAC) and the full IDT, including clinical and therapy, should collaborate on the selection of this date to be sure all services can be counted into the look-back period.

Look-back period

This is the period during which information can be gathered on a resident up to and including the ARD for input into the MDS. Although the standard look-back period under MDS 3.0 is seven days, depending on the type of assessment, the look-back or observation period can be either seven or 14 days.

The selection of the ARD should truly be a team effort involving the entire IDT. The ARD will establish the look-back period for capturing services rendered to trigger the appropriate RUG category and corresponding reimbursement. Equal consideration needs to be given to both clinical and therapy needs when evaluating the selection of the ARD to ensure capture of the most appropriate reimbursement that illustrates the most accurate picture of the services rendered to meet the resident's needs during that period of review.

Completion date

This date is the date that all information is required to be gathered and documented for an assessment. In addition, all SNF staff must sign and date, indicating that it is complete. Completion dates (see Figure 4.4) vary depending on the type of assessment.

FIGURE 4.4	MDS completion requirements

Assessment Type	Completion Requirements
Federal/OBRA and PPS assessments	No later than 14 days from the ARD
Admission assessment	The CAA completion date should be no later than 14 days from the entry date
All other comprehensive MDS assessments, annual assessment updates, SCSA, and SCPA	The CAA completion date can be no later than 14 days from the ARD
Entry tracking and death in facility tracking records	Within seven days of the event date

In addition, the *RAI User's Manual* notes an important point related to completion dates:

- *For OBRA-required comprehensive assessments, assessment completion is defined as completion of the CAA process in addition to the MDS items, meaning that the RN assessment coordinator has signed and dated both the MDS (Item Z0500) and CAA(s) (Item V0200B) completion attestations. Since a comprehensive assessment includes completion of both the MDS and the CAA process, the assessment timing requirements for a comprehensive assessment apply to both the completion of the MDS and the CAA process.*

- *For noncomprehensive and discharge assessments, assessment completion is defined as completion of the MDS only, meaning that the RN assessment coordinator has signed and dated the MDS (Item Z0500) completion attestation.*

Transmission date

This is the date that the electronic submission files are transmitted to the quality improvement evaluation system (QIES) assessment submission and processing (ASAP) system. All Medicare and Medicaid nursing facilities are required to transmit MDS records through the QIES ASAP system provided by CMS. Comprehensive assessments are required to be transmitted within 14 days of the completion date of the care plan. All other MDS assessments are required to be transmitted within 14 days of the MDS completion date. Tracking records (i.e., entry tracking and death in facility tracking) must be transmitted within 14 days of the event.

Detailed Review of Care-Related Sections of the MDS

For this section of the chapter, we will use the *RAI User's Manual* as our guide. It is important to note at this time that documentation of the symptoms, treatments, services, etc., related to items recorded on the MDS is a crucial part of the overall process. As the old adage says, "If it wasn't documented, it wasn't done!" Any time something is scored on the MDS, we are required to have the adequate documentation to support what was coded, and the documentation must be from within that look-back period.

For purposes of this book, we will only review the care-related areas of the MDS 3.0 assessment tool (see Figure 4.5). Items like Section A—Identification information, related to facility information, resident demographic, and coding the reason for the assessment, will not be reviewed. We will focus on triggers for skilled services in long-term care for review in this section of the book. Each section that follows will be titled, and the "intent" of each specific section will be taken directly from the *RAI User's Manual.*

FIGURE
4.5
Sections of the MDS 3.0

Section	Title
A	Identification Information
B	Hearing, Speech, and Vision
C	Cognitive Patterns
D	Mood
E	Behavior
F	Preferences for Customary Routine and Activities
G	Functional Status
H	Bladder and Bowel
I	Active Diagnoses
J	Health Conditions
K	Swallowing/Nutritional Status
L	Oral/Dental Status
M	Skin Conditions
N	Medications
O	Special Treatments, Procedures, and Programs
P	Restraints
Q	Participation in Assessment and Goal Setting
V	Care Assessment Area (CAA) Summary
X	Correction Request
Z	Assessment Administration

Section B—Hearing, Speech, and Vision

Intent: The intent of items in this section is to document the resident's ability to hear (with assistive hearing devices, if they are used), understand, and communicate with others and whether the resident experiences visual limitations or difficulties related to diseases common in aged persons.

This section assesses a resident's ability to make him- or herself understood. Often, the inability to hear, communicate, or see properly can be mistaken for cognitive deficits. Residents who have suffered a stroke, for example, may need additional expertise and time to determine their care needs and required resources for effective care delivery. This section can have a significant impact on supporting the need for skilled care.

Section C—Cognitive Patterns

Intent: The items in this section are intended to determine the resident's attention, orientation, and ability to register and recall new information. These items are crucial factors in many care-planning decisions.

This section assesses a resident's cognitive patterns looking at whether there is a need to conduct a brief interview for mental status (BIMS) or whether the staff can assess the resident's mental status with a staff assessment for mental status (SAMS). This decision is based on whether the resident can be understood. If the resident is rarely or never understood, a SAMS is indicated. A BIMS will assess a resident in the following three areas:

- Repetition of three words

- Temporal orientation

- Recall

The performance of a BIMS will allow any cognitive deficits to be identified. According to the *RAI User's Manual,* "When cognitive impairment is incorrectly diagnosed or missed, appropriate communication, worthwhile activities, and therapies may not be offered."

Although the BIMS is the preferred method of determining cognitive function, the RAI notes the fact that some residents are unable or unwilling to participate, so a SAMS is indicated. A SAMS will assess a resident in the following four areas:

- Short-term memory

- Long-term memory

- Memory/recall ability

- Cognitive skills for daily decision-making

Additionally, this section assesses a resident's condition related to delirium and any possible onset of mental status changes. Residents who have cognitive deficits will require additional SNF resources to meet their needs and deliver services; so, this area again has a significant impact on support of skilled needs.

Section D—Mood

Intent: The items in this section address mood distress, a serious condition that is underdiagnosed and undertreated in the nursing home and is associated with significant morbidity. It is particularly important to identify signs and symptoms of mood distress among nursing home residents because these signs and symptoms can be treatable.

This section assesses a resident's mood, not only related to depression or mood disorders, but to simply record the presence or absence of the clinical indicators of mood. Scoring of information in this section does not serve as a diagnosis of depression, for example, but only serves to document the presence or absence of the mood indicators.

Similar to the assessment of cognitive skills, this section also allows for either a resident mood interview called a Patient Health Questionnaire (PHQ-9©) or a Staff Assessment of Resident Mood (PHQ-9-OV©). The type of interview completed depends on the same criteria identified with the cognitive function testing: Can the resident be understood?

Identifying mood indicators can trigger interventions that will address mood symptoms and ensure resident safety. Residents with mood indicators will require additional staff time and interventions and may contribute to supporting skilled clinical and therapy need. In addition, signs and symptoms of depression play a role in the RUG classification with the special care high, special care low, and clinically complex categories (see Figure 4.6).

| FIGURE 4.6 | | | SNF PPS RUG–IV 66 RUG groups |

Category	ADL	Splits	RUG
Rehabilitation Plus Extensive Services			
Ultra High			
Rx 720 minutes/week minimum, at least one discipline for five days/week; second discipline may be three days/week plus tracheostomy care, ventilator/respirator, or isolation for an infectious disease while a resident	11–16		RUX
	2–10		RUL
Very High			
Rx 500 minutes/week minimum, at least one discipline for five days/week plus tracheostomy care, ventilator/respirator, or isolation for an infectious disease while a resident	11–16		RVX
	2–10		RVL
High			
Rx 325 minutes/week minimum, one discipline for five days/week plus extensive service plus tracheostomy care, ventilator/respirator, or isolation for an infectious disease while a resident	11–16		RHX
	2–10		RHL
Medium			
Rx 150 minutes/week minimum, five days/week across three disciplines plus tracheostomy care, ventilator/respirator, or isolation for an infectious disease while a resident	11–16		RMX
	2–10		RML
Low			
Rx 45 minutes/week minimum three days/week plus nursing rehabilitation, two activities for 15 minutes for six days plus tracheostomy care, ventilator/respirator, or isolation for an infectious disease while a resident	2–16		RLX

FIGURE
4.6

**SNF PPS RUG–IV
66 RUG groups (cont.)**

Category	ADL	Splits	RUG
Rehabilitation			
Ultra High			
Rx 720 minutes/week minimum, at least one for discipline five days/week; second discipline may be three days/week	11–16		RUC
	6–10		RUB
	0–5		RUA
Very High			
Rx 500 minutes/week minimum, at least one discipline for five days/week	11–16		RVC
	6–10		RVB
	0–5		RVA
High			
Rx 325 minutes/week minimum, one discipline for five days/week	11–16		RHC
	6–10		RHB
	0–5		RHA
Medium			
Rx 150 minutes/week for five days/week across three disciplines	11–16		RMC
	6–10		RMB
	0–5		RMA
Low			
Rx 45 minutes/week for a minimum of three days/week plus nursing rehabilitation; two activities for 15 minutes for six days	11–16		RLB
	0–10		RLA
Extensive Services			
Tracheostomy care **and** ventilator/respirator while a resident			ES3
Tracheostomy care **or** ventilator/respirator while a resident	2–16		ES2
Isolation for active infectious disease while a resident		Based on situation	ES1

FIGURE
4.6

**SNF PPS RUG–IV
66 RUG groups (cont.)**

Category	ADL	Splits	RUG
Special Care High			
Comatose (completely activities-of-daily-living [ADL] dependent) with septicemia; diabetes with daily injections and physician order changes on 2 or more days; quadriplegia with ADL ≥ 5; chronic obstructive pulmonary disease (COPD) and shortness of breath lying flat; fever with pneumonia, vomiting, or weight loss or tube feeding; parenteral/IV feeding; respiratory therapy for seven days	15–16	Depression	HE2
	15–16	No signs	HE1
	11–14	Depression	HD2
	11–14	No signs	HD1
	6–10	Depression	HC2
	6–10	No signs	HC1
	2–5	Depression	HB2
	2–5	No signs	HB1
Special Care Low			
Cerebral palsy, multiple sclerosis, or Parkinson's disease with ADL ≥ 5; respiratory failure and oxygen therapy while a resident; feeding tube; ulcers (two or more at stage II or one or more at stage III or IV; pressure ulcers or two or more venous/arterial ulcers; or one stage II pressure ulcer and one venous/arterial ulcer) with two or more skin care treatments; foot infection/diabetic foot ulcer/open lesions of the foot with treatment; radiation therapy while a resident; dialysis while a resident	15–16	Depression	LE2
	15–16	No signs	LE1
	11–14	Depression	LD2
	11–14	No signs	LD1
	6–10	Depression	LC2
	6–10	No signs	LC1
	2–5	Depression	LB2
	2–5	No signs	LB1

FIGURE
4.6

**SNF PPS RUG–IV
66 RUG groups (cont.)**

Category	ADL	Splits	RUG
Clinically Complex			
Extensive services, special care high or special care low qualifier with ADL of 0–1; pneumonia, hemiplegia with ADL ≥ 5; surgical wounds or open lesions with treatment; burns; chemotherapy while a resident; oxygen therapy while a resident; IV medications while a resident; transfusion while a resident	15–16	Depression	CE2
	15–16	No signs	CE1
	11–14	Depression	CD2
	11–14	No signs	CD1
	6–10	Depression	CC2
	6–10	No signs	CC1
	2–5	Depression	CB2
	2–5	No signs	CB1
	0–1	Depression	CA2
	0–1	No signs	CA1
Behavioral Symptoms and Cognitive Performance			
Cognitive impairment BIMs score ≤ 9 or cognitive performance scale ≥ 3; hallucinations, delusions; residents displaying any of the following on four or more days over the last seven days: physical or verbal behavioral symptoms toward others, other behavioral symptoms, rejection of care, or wandering; ADL score < 5	2–5	Two or more restorative nursing six or more days/week	BB2
	2–5	Less restorative	BB1
	0–1	Two or more restorative nursing six or more days/week	BA2
	0–1	Less restorative	BA1

FIGURE
4.6

**SNF PPS RUG–IV
66 RUG groups (cont.)**

Category	ADL	Splits	RUG
Reduced Physical Functioning			

Residents not qualifying for other categories
 	
Restorative nursing services include the following:
 	
    Urinary and/or bowel training program
    Passive and/or active range of motion
    Splint and/or brace assistance
    Bed mobility and/or walking training
    Transfer training
    Dressing and/or grooming training
    Eating and/or swallowing training
    Amputation/prosthesis care training
    Communication training
 	
Notes:
No clinical variables used
	15–16	Two or more restorative nursing six or more days/week	PE2

	15–16	Less restorative	PE1
	11–14	Two or more restorative nursing six or more days/week	PD2
	11–14	Less restorative	PD1
	6–10	Two or more restorative nursing six or more days/week	PC2
	6–10	Less restorative	PC1
	2–5	Two or more restorative nursing six or more days/week	PB2
	2–5	Less restorative	PB1
	0–1	Nursing rehab	PA2
	0–1	Less restorative	PA1
Default			AAA

Section E—Behavior

Intent: The items in this section identify behavioral symptoms in the last seven days that may cause distress to the resident or that may be distressing or disruptive to facility residents, staff members, or the care environment. These behaviors may place the resident at risk for injury, isolation, and inactivity and may also indicate unrecognized needs, preferences, or illness. Behaviors include those that are potentially self-harmful to the resident. The emphasis is on identifying behaviors, which does not necessarily imply a medical diagnosis. Identification of the frequency and the impact of behavioral symptoms on the resident and on others is critical to distinguish behaviors that constitute problems from those that are not problematic. Once the frequency and impact of behavioral symptoms are accurately determined, follow-up evaluation and care plan interventions can be developed to improve the symptoms or reduce their impact.

This section does not necessarily focus on the intent of the resident's actions, but rather focuses on the actions themselves. Whether the resident intended to behave a certain way is irrelevant; behavior scoring is related only to what the actions actually were. Similar to mood, addressing resident behaviors and providing the proper interventions will require staff resources and will contribute to the RUG calculation.

Section F—Preferences for Customary Routine and Activities

Intent: The intent of items in this section is to obtain information regarding the resident's preferences for his or her daily routine and activities. This is best accomplished when the information is obtained directly from the resident or through the family or significant other, or through staff interviews if the resident cannot report preferences. The information obtained during this interview is just a portion of the assessment. Nursing homes should use this as a guide to create an individualized plan based on the resident's preferences and is not meant to be all-inclusive.

Although this section of the MDS does not speak specifically to the skilled needs of the resident, it does speak toward an important initiative of MDS 3.0—Resident-centered provision of care. In the rollout of MDS 3.0, CMS wanted residents to have the ability to play a role in their care provision, which could improve their clinical outcomes and provide for more accurate information.

Section G—Functional Status

Intent: Items in this section assess the need for assistance with activities of daily living (ADL), and include such issues as altered gait, balance problems, and a decreased range of motion. In addition, on admission, resident and staff opinions regarding functional rehabilitation potential are noted.

This section of the MDS is crucial because a resident's ADL score is what differentiates RUG levels within each category. In addition, the four late-loss ADLs, which include bed mobility, transfers, eating, and toilet use are the most common areas of care needed in a long-term, skilled care setting. Proper coding of this section is crucial to identify and meet the needs of residents accurately, and is the most often undercoded section of the MDS. In addition, undercoding this section is the most common area of undercoding in a SNF. The issue is that this type of undercoding reduces reimbursement to the SNF, which the SNF is entitled to, for the additional resources and staff time it is expending to care for its residents.

That said, it is imperative to be sure the RNAC is capturing documentation from all three shifts for the seven-day look-back period in this area as most residents are most dependent in the evening or in the middle of the night. The *RAI User's Manual* offers the following guidance related to assessing a resident for Section G:

> *When reviewing records, interviewing staff, and observing the resident, be specific in evaluating each component as listed in the ADL activity definition. For example, when evaluating Bed Mobility, determine the level of assistance required for moving the resident to and from a lying position, for turning the resident from side to side, and/or for positioning the resident in bed.*

> *Coding of this section is recorded in two categories: Self Performance and Support. What did the resident do for him- or herself (self performance) and what support was provided by staff (support). The scoring of the ADL index can range from a score of 0–16; and is calculated by the RUG-IV grouper software automatically based on coding of self performance and support. There are very specific rules related to how this section is coded. For purposes of this book, we will not get into the details of coding in this section. However, it is imperative to stress the need for coding accuracy in the late-loss ADLs for proper documentation and reimbursement under Medicare Part A.*

Section H—Bladder and Bowel

Intent: The intent of the items in this section is to gather information on the use of bowel and bladder appliances, the use of and response to urinary toileting programs, urinary and bowel continence, bowel training programs, and bowel patterns. Each resident who is incontinent or at risk of developing incontinence should be identified, assessed, and provided with individualized treatment (medications, nonmedicinal treatments, and/or devices) and services to achieve or maintain as normal elimination function as possible.

This section identifies the presence of the following "appliances":

- Indwelling catheter

- External catheter

- Ostomy

- Intermittent catheterization

All of the previously listed "appliances" require more supplies and staff time, and coding of the presence of these items plays into the skilled need and reimbursement for the services provided. In addition, this section addresses urinary and bowel continence, urinary toileting programs, and bowel patterns. This area of care is common in long-term care. Properly identifying and providing services in this area can lower the risk of pressure ulcers, increase self-esteem, reduce dependence on caregivers, and reduce the cost of care.

Section I—Active Diagnoses

Intent: The items in this section are intended to code diseases that have a relationship to the resident's current functional status, cognitive status, mood or behavior status, medical treatments, nursing monitoring, or risk of death. One of the important functions of the MDS assessment is to generate an updated, accurate picture of the resident's health status.

As we have discussed earlier in the book, a resident cannot be skilled based on his or her diagnosis alone. That said, this section of the MDS can significantly impact coverage of a resident under Medicare

Part A and reimbursement for services. You will notice in Figure 4.6, the special care high, special care low, and clinically complex RUG categories all mention diagnoses such as chronic obstructive pulmonary disease (COPD), cerebral palsy, multiple sclerosis, Parkinson's disease, diabetes, and hemiplegia. Residents with these specific diagnoses can significantly impact a resident's health and require more staff time and interventions to properly care for such comorbities. The diagnosis or conditions noted in Figure 4.6 do not identify every possibility to record in Section I; rather, they may be specific RUG category triggers if active treatment related to those diagnoses occurs. Documentation of the presence of specific diagnosis or conditions is crucial to paint an overall accurate picture of a resident to properly identify the need for skilled services.

Section J—Health Conditions

Intent: The intent of the items in this section is to document a number of health conditions that impact the resident's functional status and quality of life. The items include an assessment of pain, which uses an interview with the resident or staff if the resident is unable to participate. The pain items assess the presence of pain, pain frequency, effect on function, intensity, management, and control. Other items in the section assess dyspnea, tobacco use, prognosis, problem conditions, and falls.

This section represents another section where a resident interview plays a part in the proper coding. Similar to what we discussed earlier, the resident's ability to be understood will determine if the resident will be interviewed regarding his or her pain or if the staff will identify indicators of pain or possible pain. The assessment of pain management has a five-day look-back period and focuses on the following areas:

- Pain presence

- Pain frequency

- Pain effect on function

- Pain intensity

Other areas identified in this section include shortness of breath, tobacco use, prognosis (if the resident has a condition or chronic disease that may result in a life expectancy of less then six months), problem conditions (e.g., fever, vomiting, dehydration, and internal bleeding), and history of falls. Again, all of these areas have a significant impact on staff time and resources needed to properly care for the resident and meet his or her needs and will contribute to the identification of skilled needs.

Section K—Swallowing/Nutritional Status

Intent: The items in this section are intended to assess the many conditions that could affect the resident's ability to maintain adequate nutrition and hydration. This section covers swallowing disorders, height and weight, weight loss, and nutritional approaches. Nurse assessors should collaborate with the dietitian and dietary staff to ensure that items in this section have been assessed and calculated accurately.

A resident's swallowing function and nutritional status is one area that creates anxiety and demands significant staff time. Per the *RAI User's Manual*:

- *The ability to swallow safely can be affected by many disease processes and functional decline.*

- *Alterations in the ability to swallow can result in choking and aspiration, which can increase the resident's risk for malnutrition, dehydration, and aspiration pneumonia.*

This section also records a resident's height and weight for purposes of documenting weight management, be it obesity, malnutrition, and/or weight loss. The last part of this section addresses nutritional approaches to identify parenteral/or IV feeding, a feeding tube, a mechanically altered diet, and/or a therapeutic diet. There is further detail required in this section to identify the proportion of total caloric and fluid intake via artificial route (i.e., feeding tube).

Residents who meet the 26%–50% of calories and 501cc of fluid per day via the feeding tube or who receive 51% or more of calories via the feeding tube during the last seven days will automatically qualify for Medicare Part A benefits in a SNF. Additionally, they are required to continue on Medicare to use a full 100-day benefit period until they drop below such levels on an MDS. These levels will also continue that spell of illness and prevent the resident from attaining the 60-day period of wellness, discussed in Chapter 2, to qualify for a new 100-day benefit period.

Section L—Oral/Dental Status

Intent: This item is intended to record any dental problems present in the seven-day look-back period.

Section M—Skin Conditions

Intent: The items in this section document the risk, presence, appearance, and change of pressure ulcers. This section also notes other skin ulcers, wounds, or lesions, and documents some treatment categories related to skin injury or avoiding injury. It is important to recognize and evaluate each resident's risk factors and to identify and evaluate all areas at risk of constant pressure. A complete assessment of skin is essential to an effective pressure ulcer prevention and skin treatment program. Be certain to include in the assessment process a holistic approach. It is imperative to determine the etiology of all wounds and lesions, as this will determine and direct the proper treatment and management of the wound.

The number of pressure ulcers, their stage, and frequency of treatment are all components of identifying a skilled need related to a skin condition. The following criteria will categorize a resident in a special care low category, provided that two or more skin care treatments, as follows, have been delivered:

- Two or more stage II pressure ulcers

- One or more stage III or IV pressure ulcers

- One stage II pressure ulcer and one venous/arterial ulcer

Again, the old adage, "You never down-stage a wound," comes into play here, which is why two or more skin treatments are required to code any pressure ulcers in this section for skilled coverage. In addition to pressure ulcers, the presence of other ulcers, wounds, and skin problems are also documented in this section as they may identify a resident who is at risk for further skin complications or the development of pressure ulcers. However, some of the additional wound care services may categorize the resident into a clinically complex category and not special care high, such as surgical wounds and open lesions with treatment.

This is another area that is relatively cut and dry related to the provision of skilled services. If you are providing wound care, working with open lesions or surgical wounds, you are most likely providing a skilled service.

Section N—Medications

Intent: The intent of the items in this section is to record the number of days, during the last seven days (or since admission/reentry if less than seven days), that any type of injection, insulin, and/or select oral medications were received by the resident.

Monitor the number of injections and medications you administer to a resident. This quantity serves as a reminder to staff to monitor adverse consequences and medication order changes. For example, a diagnosis of diabetes with daily injections and physician order changes on two or more days could qualify a resident for Medicare Part A coverage under the special care high category.

Section O—Special Treatments, Procedures, and Programs

Intent: The intent of the items in this section is to identify any special treatments, procedures, and programs that the resident received during the specified times. This section identifies provision of the following special treatments, procedures, and programs in the last 14 days:

- Chemotherapy

- Radiation

- Oxygen therapy

- Suctioning (tracheal and/or nasopharyngeal suctioning only; not oral suctioning)

- Tracheostomy care

- Ventilator or respirator

- BiPAP/CPAP

- IV medications

- Transfusions

- Dialysis

- Hospice care

- Respite care

- Isolation or quarantine for active infectious disease

However, SNFs are cautioned that coding any of the previous items that were performed in conjunction with a surgical or diagnostic procedure is not allowed. These services are further distinguished depending on when they are provided. Prior to admission/entry into the SNF and after admission/entry into the SNF and when the service was provided will have a direct impact on whether the service constitutes a skilled need.

When coding isolation or quarantine for active infectious disease, the *RAI User's Manual* further clarifies:

> *Code only when the resident requires strict isolation or quarantine alone in a separate room because of active infection (i.e., symptomatic and/or have a positive test and are in the contagious stage) with a communicable disease, in an attempt to prevent spread of illness. Do not code this item if the resident only has a history of infectious disease (e.g., MRSA or C-Diff with no active symptoms), but facility policy requires cohorting of similar infectious disease conditions. Do not code this item if the "isolation" primarily consists of body/fluid precautions, because these types of precautions apply to everyone.*

This section also requires the documentation of the influenza and pneumococcal vaccines.

Another item coded in Section O is therapy services. As identified in Figure 4.6, the provision of therapy services represents a stand-alone skilled need based on the number of minutes provided, the therapy discipline, and the frequency of treatments. However, therapy needs, combined with clinical needs, can qualify a resident into the rehab plus extensive services categories as well.

Minutes provided in speech-language pathology (SLP), occupational therapy (OT), and physical therapy (PT) are broken out by the minutes provided and the number of days that the services were provided.

Therapy minutes are further broken out by the number of individual minutes, the number of concurrent minutes, and the number of group therapy minutes. All therapy minutes and days are recorded using a seven-day look-back period. Definitions of each type of therapy and any limitations are as follows:

- Individual therapy represents the total minutes the resident received one-on-one treatment

- Concurrent therapy represents the total minutes the resident received treatment concurrently with one other resident (cannot exceed 50% of total minutes)

- Group therapy represents the total minutes the resident received treatment as part of a group of residents (cannot exceed 25% of total minutes)

Therapy minutes documented on the MDS should only include actual treatment time, not time spent on the evaluation or documentation. Therapy minutes cannot be projected for purposes of Section O; only minutes actually delivered during the look-back period can be counted. Days of therapy is recorded as the number of days in the seven day look-back period that the resident received at least 15 minutes of treatment.

The RUG categories for rehab or rehab plus extensive services are further broken down by the number of disciplines treating the resident and how many days per week the resident received the treatments. Additional therapies, such as respiratory therapy, psychological therapy, and recreational therapy are also coded in Section O.

The second to last item documented in Section O is restorative nursing interventions. The *RAI User's Manual* states the following:

- *Restorative nursing program refers to nursing interventions that promote the resident's ability to adapt and adjust to living as independently and safely as possible. This concept actively focuses on achieving and maintaining optimal physical, mental, and psychosocial functioning.*

- *A resident may be started on a restorative nursing program when he or she is admitted to the facility with restorative needs, but is not a candidate for formalized rehabilitation therapy, or when restorative needs arise during the course of a longer-term stay, or in conjunction with formalized rehabilitation therapy. Generally, restorative nursing programs are initiated when a resident is discharged from formalized physical, occupational, or speech rehabilitation therapy.*

Examples of restorative nursing programs include the following:

- Passive and/or active range of motion

- Splint or brace assistance

- Bed mobility

- Transfer

- Walking

- Dressing and/or grooming

- Eating and/or swallowing

- Amputation/prosthetic care

- Communication

The final item documented in Section O is physician order changes. How many times during the last 14 days did the resident receive physician order changes? This is a crucial component as frequent order changes can trigger coverage in some of the clinical categories, with the presence of other triggers.

Section P—Restraints

Intent: The intent of this section is to record the frequency over the seven-day look-back period that the resident was restrained by any of the listed devices at any time during the day or night. Assessors will evaluate whether a device meets the definition of a physical restraint and will code only the devices that meet the definition in the appropriate categories of Item P0100.

Although restraint use does not, by itself, constitute a skilled need, it is used by CMS in monitoring its commitment to reduce unnecessary physical restraints in nursing homes and ensuring residents are not being restrained unless it is deemed necessary and appropriate as determined by the regulation.

Section Q—Participation in Assessment and Goal Setting

Intent: The items in this section are intended to record the participation and expectations of the resident, family members, or significant other(s) in the assessment, and to understand the resident's overall goals.

Again, although this section does not necessarily contribute to the assessment of a skilled need, it is nonetheless an important piece of the assessment process.

Overwhelmed?

Let us slow it down and regroup. All of the rules and regulations discussed in Chapters 2 and 3 are discussed in further detail in the *RAI User's Manual* and broken down into exact services provided to residents in a section-by-section format. Each type of service, procedure, or treatment is separated by a section. Each section then further delineates all of the possible components that can contribute to the skilled needs of residents and assists SNF staff in identifying and documenting such items.

There are four main reasons why we fail to skill residents consistently under Medicare Part A:

- Lack of knowledge of the rules and regulations

- Desire to not be challenged by a Medicare reviewer

- Documentation in the medical record may not be supportive

- The MDS is inaccurately coded and creates a picture of a nonskilled resident

If you can get a handle on these four roadblocks to accurately identify skilled needs of SNF residents, you will be able to assist your residents in using the benefit they are entitled to, provide exceptional care that meets all of your residents' needs, and be reimbursed according to the services provided.

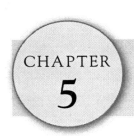

Proper Communication During a Medicare Part A Stay

We have certainly covered a lot of ground in Chapters 1 through 4; now we come to the point where we need to make sure skilled nursing facility (SNF) staff are constantly communicating with each other. This communication needs to cover continued Medicare Part A services, proper documentation of those services, and ending Medicare Part A services.

The Medicare Meeting

What is the purpose of the Medicare meeting? This meeting allows the interdisciplinary team (IDT) to review each resident and discuss his or her individual needs related to the skilled services being provided. It also allows for the opportunity to improve resident outcomes through a coordinated system of care delivery. Before we begin reviewing what should be covered during the Medicare meeting, let us discuss who should attend the meeting and how often the meeting should be held.

Who should attend the Medicare meeting?

At a minimum, the following IDT members should be present for the meeting:

- Registered nurse assessment coordinator (RNAC)

- Therapy representative

- Nursing representative

- Social services

- Accounting/billing

- Medical records

- May include other direct line staff, if needed, to discuss specific resident care concerns

How often should the meeting be held?

The Medicare meeting should occur at least weekly from a formal meeting perspective. However, many SNFs, depending on their utilization, hold a daily "stand-up" meeting to review the daily activities or items, and then hold a more formal weekly Medicare meeting where residents are discussed in greater detail.

What preparation should be completed prior to the meeting?

The following information, for example, should be prepared or reviewed by each department, where applicable:

- Nursing

  - Current medical status of resident to include, but not limited to, falls, infections, cognition, mobility, feeding, weight loss, diagnosis, medication changes, and tests performed

  - Family concerns

  - Skilled nursing services provided to date and planned interventions

  - Recent or scheduled physician visits

  - Anticipated needs or changes that may affect the care plan

  - Discharge plan

  - Nursing notes

- Therapy (by discipline)

  - Functional status

  - Skilled interventions and resident progress

  - Level of resident participation

  - Equipment needs

  - Discharge plan

  - Therapy notes

- Social services

  - Anticipated discharge location and support structure

  - Family concerns

  - Review of social service notes

- Minimum data set (MDS)

  - Next assessment reference date (ARD)

  - Current and anticipated next resource utilization group (RUG) level

  - Other Medicare Required Assessments (OMRA)/start of therapy (SOT) and/or end of therapy (EOT) assessments

  - Signatures needed on completed MDSs

  - Discrepancies

- Medical records

  - Missing or incomplete therapy plans of treatment

  - Missing or incomplete physician certifications and recertifications

  - Medical and treatment diagnosis

- Accounting/billing

  - Number of Medicare Part A days used

  - Ancillary charges

Meeting and agenda

Each resident record should be reviewed in detail. Often, this is also a good venue to multitask and perform a "triple check."

A triple check is a necessary component of any successful SNF Medicare program. Each SNF may have small variances on what is referred to as the triple check, but essentially it is verifying information between admissions, clinical, therapy, and billing before any claims are submitted.

The triple check is discussed later in this chapter.

FIGURE
5.1

Resident services meeting record

Resident Name: _____ MR#: _____ Meeting Date: _____

☐ M/C A   Medicare Days Used: _____ as of _____   Medical Diagnosis: _____

Current RUG Level _____   Next ARD Window: From _____ to _____   Proposed ARD _____

Anticipated RUG level: _____   Scheduled Assessments: Significant Change: ☐ Yes ☐ No Date: _____

☐ 3-day qualifying hospital stay verified   OMRA: ☐ Yes ☐ No Date: _____

☐ M/C B   ☐ HMO _____   ☐ Private _____   ☐ Other: _____

First Medicare Meeting Only: Verify diagnosis codes on the MDS match the codes input into claims software.

Verified by Medicare Team: ☐ Yes   ☐ No

Nursing Services: *See nurses notes and care plan in the medical record.

Since the last meeting, resident has received the following services:

Physician Office Visit(s): ☐ Yes ☐ No Date: _____   X-Ray/Lab: ☐ Yes ☐ No   Supplies: ☐ Yes ☐ No

Overall condition: ☐ Improving   ☐ Stable   ☐ Declining

Changes/updates:

Therapy Services: ☐ PT   ☐ OT   ☐ Speech   ☐ Dysphagia

*See therapy evaluation, plan of care and daily note in Medical Record.

Overall condition: ☐ Improving   ☐ Stable   ☐ Declining

Changes/updates:

Additional Concerns/Issues/Requests:

FIGURE	
5.1	**Resident services meeting record (cont.)**

Due to the continued need for skilled services on a daily basis, Medicare A coverage will continue: ☐ Yes ☐ No

Discharge Planning: Anticipated discharge time frame: _____

Anticipated Discharge Location: ☐ Residential   ☐ Assisted   ☐ Catered   ☐ Off-campus   ☐ Remain in facility

Level of Support Available: _____

Wellness Program referral: ☐ Yes ☐ No   Home assessment needed: ☐ Yes ☐ No   Family training needed: ☐ Yes ☐ No

Equipment needed: ☐ Yes   ☐ No   If yes, list_____

Signatures/Date:

_____   _____

_____   _____

Source: Covenant Retirement Communities. Used with permission.

Figure 5.1 is an example of a very comprehensive resident services meeting record; you will note that this form also includes "Medicare Part B," "HMO," "Private," and "Other" in the discussion points. This form is an example of a record that could be used for all payer types, but can also be adapted to only serve as a tool used to review Medicare Part A residents. The two clinical areas of nursing and therapy should be discussed separately, and with equal weight given to each to properly identify all services being provided to the resident. Often, when therapy services are coming to an end, SNF staff forget about the clinical services the resident is receiving and may continue to receive after therapy services end.

As we reviewed in Chapter 4, there are four categories of RUGs that are strictly clinical in nature: extensive services, special care high, special care low, and clinically complex. It is imperative that the residents' clinical needs be given just as much consideration as any rehabilitation needs. Using the Medicare meeting as a venue for all disciplines is critical to the success of your Medicare program. Although this next statement is a hot topic of debate at times, the leader of the Medicare meeting should be the RNAC, not therapy or billing. The RNAC is responsible for the coordination of the MDS, care area assessments (CAA), and care plan, so it makes sense to have the RNAC facilitate the Medicare meeting.

That said, let us move on to review what should be covered in a Medicare meeting in greater detail.

Admissions/demographic information review

First of all, resident information should be verified, including demographic information, prior Medicare Part A days used, and confirmation of the three-day qualifying hospital stay. Another important component of the admissions information review is the admitting diagnosis codes. As we discussed earlier in Chapter 3, the Medicare Part A SNF care has to be rendered for a condition for which the patient received inpatient hospital services or for a condition that arose while receiving care in a SNF for a condition for which he or she received inpatient hospital services.

Ensuring that the admitting diagnosis is traceable back to the reason for hospitalization is a crucial piece of the intricate puzzle. The next step is to ensure that diagnoses from both nursing and therapy are also reflected in the MDS and in the software used for admissions, billing, and/or claims management.

MDS and assessments

An important component of this meeting is to discuss current assessments, including making sure all staff involved are aware of the upcoming assessments and discussing the need for any off-cycle assessments such as an OMRA, SOT, EOT, or significant changes in status assessment (SCSA). At this time, the next ARD window should be discussed for any off-cycle or regularly scheduled assessments to ensure that all staff involved are aware of the look-back period for the next MDS.

Nursing information review

At this time, the actual clinical chart should be reviewed. As indicated previously, the expectation is that a nurse representative has prepared for the meeting and can provide a synopsis for the group on what is happening with the resident from a nursing perspective. Items discussed should include a resident's functional status, medications, treatments, other skilled services being rendered, special tests, or physician visit updates … just to name a few!

Therapy information review

If the resident is receiving therapy services, those services should be discussed in detail as well. One representative from therapy should be present at all meetings; it is not necessary to have a physical therapist, occupational therapist, and speech-language pathologist attend every meeting. Often, the manager of the therapy department will attend and speak for the group on each resident, as he or she has been briefed by the other therapy staff prior to the meeting. Each therapy discipline should be discussed in detail related to resident progress and current level of function. Special attention should be paid to making sure that the nursing documentation and therapy documentation are painting a similar resident picture; if it is not, that issue needs to be addressed at this meeting.

Other departments

Social services should be prepared to discuss the ongoing discharge plan for the resident and update the team on any decisions that will be made on whether the resident will be remaining in the nursing home long term, or returning to his or her home or to a family member's home. If the resident is expected to discharge out of the SNF, it is a good time to discuss what level of support the resident is going to need and what level of support will be available to him or her in the home setting. Therapy may also need to work on some additional areas such as car transfers or performing a home visit to identify any adjustment to the environment or possible equipment needs to assist with the resident's transition to the home setting. It is also important to discuss the anticipated Medicare Part A discharge time frame because proper notice will be required prior to ending skilled services. This is discussed in more detail later in this chapter.

Medical Records should report on whether the necessary signatures have been properly obtained and if all orders are present and accounted for related to services that the resident is receiving. For example, physician signatures are needed on the physician certification and recertification forms, and therapist and physician signatures are needed on the therapy plans of treatment.

The group should then make a collective decision on whether the resident will continue receiving Medicare Part A skilled services or whether a discharge is looming.

Ending Medicare Part A Skilled Services

According to the Centers for Medicare & Medicaid Services (CMS), both Medicare beneficiaries and providers have certain rights and protections related to financial liability under the fee-for-service (FFS)

Medicare and the Medicare Advantage (MA) programs. These financial liability and appeal rights and protections are communicated to beneficiaries through notices given by providers.

Expedited review

Beginning July 1, 2005, any time a SNF will be ending skilled services under either Medicare Part A or Medicare Part B, a formal notice to the beneficiary is required. The new process that was introduced is called the expedited review process. The SNF is required to provide the beneficiary with a generic notice (see Figure 5.2). The generic notice informs the beneficiary that skilled services are ending and informs them of their right to appeal to the quality improvement organization (QIO) for their state or region. The detailed notice (see Figure 5.3) is issued if the beneficiary requests a review from the QIO and provides more detailed information about the services the resident was receiving and the reason for the termination of services generic notice. The generic notice simply states that skilled services will be ending on the specific date and that the resident has the right to appeal the decision to terminate services with the QIO, with QIO contact information provided. The generic notice must be issued no later than two days prior to the termination of skilled services, per *42 CFR §405.1200(b)*. The CMS instructions for the notice indicate that the notice must be "validly delivered." This refers not only to delivering the notice in complete form and in a timely manner, but also to providers who are required to be sure that the resident understands the purpose and information in the notice for the delivery to be valid. In the case, where the resident is unable to sign for him- or herself, the notice should be delivered to the resident's representative. The following is the procedure to be followed if a resident is unable to sign:

- If the provider is unable to personally deliver a notice of noncoverage to a person legally acting on behalf of a beneficiary, then the provider should telephone the representative to advise him or her when the beneficiary's services are no longer covered.

- The beneficiary's appeal rights must be explained to the representative, and the name and telephone number of the appropriate QIO should be provided.

- The date of the conversation is the date of the receipt of the notice. Confirm the telephone contact by written notice mailed on that same date.

- Place a dated copy of the notice in the beneficiary's medical file and document the telephone contact to include the name of the person initiating the contact, the name of the representative contacted, the date and time of the contact, and the telephone number called.

- When direct phone contact cannot be made, send the notice to the representative by certified mail, with a return receipt requested.

- The date that someone at the representative's address signs (or refuses to sign) the receipt is the date of receipt.

- When notices are returned by the post office, with no indication of a refusal date, then the beneficiary's liability starts on the second working day after the provider's mailing date.

These procedures also may be used where a beneficiary has authorized or appointed an individual to act on his or her behalf, and the provider cannot obtain the signature of the beneficiary's representative through direct personal contact.

Detailed notice

The detailed notice is issued when the resident or the resident's representative requests a review by the QIO, after receipt of the generic notice to allow the third party (QIO) to review the resident's records and either agrees or disagrees with the decision to terminate skilled services. The detailed notice must be issued no later than end of business on the day that the QIO issues the notification of the resident request, per *42 CFR §405.1202(f)(1)*. This notice reiterates the date of termination, but also goes into additional detail surrounding:

1. Facts used to make the decision. This is where the provider will fill in the patient-specific detail of why the services are ending.

2. Detailed explanation of why the services are no longer covered under Medicare. This is where the provider will relate the patient-specific reasons for termination to the Medicare rules that support the decision being made.

Detailed completion instructions for both the generic and detailed notices can be found on the Beneficiary Notification Initiative section of the CMS website. If the resident will be remaining in the SNF receiving nonskilled care, an advanced beneficiary notice (ABN) will be required and is discussed in the next section.

FIGURE
5.2

Generic notice

OMB Approval No. 0938-0953

{Insert logo here}
NOTICE OF MEDICARE PROVIDER NON-COVERAGE

Patient Name: **Patient ID Number:**

THE EFFECTIVE DATE COVERAGE OF YOUR CURRENT {insert type}
SERVICES WILL END: **{insert effective date}**

- Your provider has determined that Medicare probably will not pay for your current {insert type} services after the effective date indicated above.
- You may have to pay for any {insert type} services you receive after the above date.

YOUR RIGHT TO APPEAL THIS DECISION

- You have the right to an immediate, independent medical review (appeal), while your services continue, of the decision to end Medicare coverage of these services.
- If you choose to appeal, the independent reviewer will ask for your opinion and you should be available to answer questions or supply information. The reviewer will also look at your medical records and/or other relevant information. You do not have to prepare anything in writing, but you have the right to do so if you wish.
- If you choose to appeal, you and the independent reviewer will each receive a copy of the detailed explanation about why your coverage for services should not continue. You will receive this detailed notice only after you request an appeal.
- If you choose to appeal, and the independent reviewer agrees that services should no longer be covered after the effective date indicated above, Medicare will not pay for these services after that date.
- If you stop services no later than the effective date indicated above, you will avoid financial liability.

HOW TO ASK FOR AN IMMEDIATE APPEAL

- You must make your request to your Quality Improvement Organization (also known as a QIO). A QIO is the independent reviewer authorized by Medicare to review the decision to end these services.
- Your request for an immediate appeal should be made as soon as possible, but no later than noon of the day before the effective date indicated above.
- The QIO will notify you of its decision as soon as possible, generally by no later than two days after the effective date of this notice.
- Call your QIO at: {insert name and number of QIO} to appeal, or if you have questions.

See page 2 of this form for more information.

FIGURE

5.2

Generic notice (cont.)

OTHER APPEAL RIGHTS:

- If you miss the deadline for filing an immediate appeal, you may still be able to file an appeal with a QIO, but the QIO will take more time to make its decision.
- Contact 1-800-MEDICARE (1-800-633-4227), or TTY: 1-877-486-2048 for more information about the appeals process.

ADDITIONAL INFORMATION (OPTIONAL)

Please sign below to indicate that you have received this notice.

I have been notified that coverage of my services will end on the effective date indicated on this notice and that I may appeal this decision by contacting my QIO.

_____

Signature of Patient or Representative

_____

Date

Form No. CMS-10123   Exp. Date 07/31/2011

According to the Paperwork Reduction Act of 1995, no persons are required to respond to a collection of information unless it displays a valid OMB control number. The valid OMB control number for this information collection is 0938-0953. The time required to prepare and distribute this collection is 10 minutes per notice, including the time to select the preprinted form, complete it and deliver it to the beneficiary. If you have comments concerning the accuracy of the time estimates or suggestions for improving this form, please write to CMS, PRA Clearance Officer, 7500 Security Boulevard, Baltimore, Maryland 21244-1850.

Detailed notice

OMB Approval No. 0938-0953

{Insert Logo here}

DETAILED EXPLANATION OF [Insert type] NON-COVERAGE

Date:

Patient Name: Patient ID Number:

This notice gives a detailed explanation of why your provider has determined that Medicare coverage for your current {insert type} services should end. ***This notice is not the decision on your appeal.*** The decision on your appeal will come from your Quality Improvement Organization (QIO).

We have reviewed your case and decided that Medicare coverage of your current {insert type} services should end.

- **The facts used to make this decision:**

- **Detailed explanation of why these services are no longer covered, and the specific Medicare coverage rules and policy used to make this decision:**

If you would like a copy of the policy or coverage guidelines used to make this decision, or a copy of the documents sent to the QIO, please call us at {insert provider telephone number}:

Form No. CMS-10124   Exp. Date 07/31/2011

Other Notification Requirements

There may also be times during a resident's Medicare Part A stay that other formal notice will be required. We will now review some of those additional notices.

ABN

Before a SNF can furnish any items or services, or before an item or service is reduced or terminated, the SNF is required to notify the beneficiary of the fact that the SNF does not expect Medicare to pay for an item or service. SNFs have the option of using the published ABN, or one of the five SNF denial letters. We will discuss use of the ABN for purposes of this book, but the denial letter paragraphs can be found in Chapter 30 of the *Claims Processing Manual*, Section 70.4.5. There are currently two ABNs that apply to SNF services.

- SNFABN–CMS–10055 (SNF Medicare Part A services only; see Figure 5.4)

- ABN–CMS–R-131 (SNF Medicare Part B services only; see Figure 5.5)

It is also important to note that CMS has been in the process of developing a revised SNFABN to replace both of the previously referenced forms to be used for either Medicare Part A or Medicare Part B services in a SNF. As of the date of publication of this book, that draft copy had not been approved and provided for use. When the revised SNFABN is approved, it will replace both the ABN–CMS–R-131 and the SNFABN–CMS–10055 for SNF providers.

FIGURE
5.4

Skilled Nursing Facility Advance Beneficiary Notice (SNFABN)

SKILLED NURSING FACILITY'S NAME & ADDRESS
TELEPHONE NO. AND TTYTDD NO.

Skilled Nursing Facility Advance Beneficiary Notice (SNFABN)

Date of Notice:_____

NOTE: You need to make a choice about receiving these health care items or services.

It is not Medicare's opinion, but our opinion, that Medicare will not pay for the item(s) or service(s) described below. Medicare does not pay for all of your health care costs. Medicare only pays for covered items and services when Medicare rules are met. The fact that Medicare may not pay for a particular item or service does not mean that you should not receive it. There may be a good reason to receive it. Right now, in your case, **Medicare probably will not pay for –**

Items or Services:

Because:

The purpose of this form is to help you make an informed choice about whether or not you want to receive these items or services, knowing that you might have to pay for them yourself. Before you make a decision about your options, you should **read this entire notice carefully**.

- Ask us to explain, if you don't understand why Medicare probably won't pay.
- Ask us how much these items or services will cost you (**Estimated Cost: $_____**), in case you have to pay for them yourself or through other insurance you may have. Your other insurance is:_____
- If in 90 days you have not gotten a decision on your claim, contact the Medicare contractor at: Address:_____
  _____ or at: Telephone: _____ TTY/TDD:_____.
- If you receive these items or services, we will submit your claim for them to Medicare.

PLEASE CHOOSE **ONE** OPTION. CHECK **ONE** BOX. **DATE & SIGN** THIS NOTICE.

☐ **Option 1. YES. I want to receive these items or services.** I understand that Medicare will not decide whether to pay unless I receive these items or services. I understand you will notify me when my claim is submitted and that you will not bill me for these items or services until Medicare makes its decision. If Medicare denies payment, I agree to be personally and fully responsible for payment. That is, I will pay personally, either out of pocket or through any other insurance that I have. I understand that I can appeal Medicare's decision.

☐ **Option 2. NO. I will not receive these items or services.** I understand that you will not be able to submit a claim to Medicare and that I will not be able to appeal your opinion that Medicare won't pay. I understand that, in the case of any physician-ordered items or services, I should notify my doctor who ordered them that I did not receive them.

Patient's Name:_____ Medicare # (HICN):_____

_____   _____
Date   Signature of the patient or of the authorized representative

FIGURE 5.5	Advance Beneficiary Notice of Noncoverage (ABN)

(A) Notifier(s):
(B) Patient Name: _____ **(C)** Identification Number: _____

ADVANCE BENEFICIARY NOTICE OF NONCOVERAGE (ABN)

<u>NOTE</u>: If Medicare doesn't pay for **(D)**_____ below, you may have to pay.

Medicare does not pay for everything, even some care that you or your health care provider have good reason to think you need. We expect Medicare may not pay for the **(D)**_____ below.

(D)_____	**(E)** Reason Medicare May Not Pay:	**(F)** Estimated Cost:

WHAT YOU NEED TO DO NOW:

- Read this notice, so you can make an informed decision about your care.
- Ask us any questions that you may have after you finish reading.
- Choose an option below about whether to receive the **(D)**_____ listed above.
  Note: If you choose Option 1 or 2, we may help you to use any other insurance that you might have, but Medicare cannot require us to do this.

(G) OPTIONS: Check only one box. We cannot choose a box for you.

❏ **OPTION 1.** I want the **(D)**_____ listed above. You may ask to be paid now, but I also want Medicare billed for an official decision on payment, which is sent to me on a Medicare Summary Notice (MSN). I understand that if Medicare doesn't pay, I am responsible for payment, but **I can appeal to Medicare** by following the directions on the MSN. If Medicare does pay, you will refund any payments I made to you, less co-pays or deductibles.

❏ **OPTION 2.** I want the **(D)**_____ listed above, but do not bill Medicare. You may ask to be paid now as I am responsible for payment. **I cannot appeal if Medicare is not billed.**

❏ **OPTION 3.** I don't want the **(D)**_____ listed above. I understand with this choice I am **not** responsible for payment, and **I cannot appeal to see if Medicare would pay.**

(H) Additional Information:

This notice gives our opinion, not an official Medicare decision. If you have other questions on this notice or Medicare billing, call **1-800-MEDICARE** (1-800-633-4227/**TTY**: 1-877-486-2048).

Signing below means that you have received and understand this notice. You also receive a copy.

(I) Signature:	**(J) Date:**

According to the Paperwork Reduction Act of 1995, no persons are required to respond to a collection of information unless it displays a valid OMB control number. The valid OMB control number for this information collection is 0938-0566. The time required to complete this information collection is estimated to average 7 minutes per response, including the time to review instructions, search existing data resources, gather the data needed, and complete and review the information collection. If you have comments concerning the accuracy of the time estimate or suggestions for improving this form, please write to: CMS, 7500 Security Boulevard, Attn: PRA Reports Clearance Officer, Baltimore, Maryland 21244-1850.

Form CMS-R-131 (03/08)   Form Approved OMB No. 0938-0566

SNFABN–CMS–10055

Per §70.1 of Chapter 30 of the *Medicare Claims Processing Manual*:

A SNFABN is a CMS-approved model written notice that the SNF gives to a Medicare beneficiary, or to her or his authorized representative, before extended care services or items are furnished, reduced, or terminated when the SNF, the UR entity, the QIO, or the Medicare contractor believes that Medicare will not pay for, or will not continue to pay for, extended care services that the SNF furnishes and that a physician ordered on the basis of one of the following statutory exclusions:

- *Not reasonable and necessary ("medical necessity") for the diagnosis or treatment of illness, injury, or to improve the functioning of a malformed body member - §1862(a)(1); or*

- *Custodial care ("not a covered level of care") - §1862(a)(9).*

A good example of when a SNFABN would be issued is if a resident is ending his or her Medicare Part A stay and will remain in the facility as a nonskilled resident. In that example, an ABN is required to be issued. A good example of when a SNFABN would not be issued is if a resident does not meet one of the technical requirements for SNF Medicare Part A coverage (i.e., three-day qualifying hospital stay). In that example, an ABN should not be issued.

ABN–CMS–R–131

This form was introduced in March 2009 and replaced the following forms:

- ABN–G (CMS–R-131-G)

- ABN–l (CMS–R-131-L)

- Notice of Exclusion from Medicare Benefits (NEMB) (CMS–20007)

The NEMB was the only form used in a SNF related to Medicare Part B services; the other forms were used for non-SNF providers. The following situations require mandatory issuance by the SNF:

- Services are not reasonable and necessary

- Custodial care

- Hospice patient who is not terminally ill

Voluntary issuances of the form can be as follows:

- Care that does not meet the definition of a Medicare benefit

- Care that is explicitly excluded from coverage (e.g., personal comfort items)

There are currently three events that could trigger the issuance of an ABN (either under Medicare Part A or Medicare Part B):

1. **Initiation**—Start of services or delivery of items that the SNF feels would not be covered. An example might be additional therapy services beyond the established goals. Medicare will only allow a provider to return a resident back to his or her prior level of functioning. If a resident has returned to that level, but wants to continue therapy to be able to walk the stairs from the lobby of the SNF to the penthouse for example, such services may not be reasonable and necessary and would require issuance of a CMS–R-131 prior to initiation.

2. **Reduction**—Decrease in a component of the current care being provided. An example may be if a beneficiary is currently receiving therapy services five days per week and the provider wishes to decrease the therapy to three days per week (please see physician order box).

3. **Termination**—Discontinuation of an item or service.

> If the physician has ordered the reduction or termination of services, there is no requirement for the SNF to issue a CMS–R-131 as the notice is not required in this situation per Chapter 30 of the *Medicare Claims Processing Manual*.

Once the resident is notified, he or she will have three options to choose from related to the identified items or services:

- *OPTION 1. I want the (D)_____ listed above. You may ask to be paid now, but I also want Medicare billed for an official decision on payment, which is sent to me on a Medicare Summary Notice (MSN). I understand that if Medicare doesn't pay, I am responsible for payment, but I can appeal to Medicare by following the directions on the MSN. If Medicare does pay, you will refund any payments I made to you, less co-pays or deductibles.*

- *OPTION 2. I want the (D)_____ listed above, but do not bill Medicare. You may ask to be paid now as I am responsible for payment. I cannot appeal if Medicare is not billed.*

- *OPTION 3. I do not want the (D)_____ listed above. I understand with this choice I am not responsible for payment, and I cannot appeal to see if Medicare would pay.*

Please review Chapter 30 of the *Medicare Claims Processing Manual* for detailed instructions on valid delivery of an ABN in both instances discussed previously.

Are there any instances when the Notice of Exclusions from Medicare Benefits (NEMB) is still used? Although the NEMB is no longer a required form, as it was replaced by the CMS–R-131, SNFs are allowed to voluntarily issue the form in cases such as the resident not meeting the technical requirements for SNF coverage, for example. However, be cautioned that use of this form allows the resident to request a billing be submitted to Medicare for a formal decision. This can cause a delay in cash flow until Medicare makes the decision. Although this is a good communication tool, SNFs can develop their own tool to communicate with residents about certain situations, such as not meeting the technical requirements for coverage without providing the option to request a bill be submitted to Medicare (see Figure 5.6).

FIGURE
5.6

**Notice of Exclusions from Medicare Benefits
Skilled Nursing Facility (NEMB-SNF)**

Notice of Exclusions from Medicare Benefits
Skilled Nursing Facility (NEMB-SNF)

Date of Notice:_____

NOTE: You need to make a choice about receiving these health care items or services.

It is not Medicare's opinion, but our opinion, that Medicare will not pay for the item(s) or service(s) described below. Medicare does not pay for all of your health care costs. Medicare only pays for covered items and services when Medicare rules are met. The fact that Medicare will not pay for a particular item or service does not mean that you should not receive it. There may be a good reason to receive it. Right now, in your case, **Medicare will not pay for –**

Items or Services:

We believe that Medicare will not pay, for the following reason. (See the reason checked off below.)

- ❏ No qualifying 3-day inpatient hospital stay.
- ❏ No days left in this benefit period.
- ❏ Care not ordered or certified by a physician.
- ❏ Daily skilled care not needed.
- ❏ SNF transfer requirement not met.
- ❏ Facility/Bed not certified by Medicare.
- ❏ Care not given by, nor supervised by, skilled nursing or rehabilitation staff.
- ❏ Items or services not furnished under arrangements by the skilled nursing facility.
- ❏ Other:_____
  _____

The purpose of this notice is to help you make an informed choice about whether or not you want to receive these items or services, knowing that you will have to pay for them yourself or through other insurance that you may have. Before you make a decision about your options, you should **read this entire notice carefully.**

- Ask us to explain, if you don't understand why Medicare won't pay.
- Ask us how much these items or services will cost you (**Estimated Cost: $_____**).
  Your other insurance is:_____

PLEASE CHOOSE ONE OPTION. CHECK ONE BOX. SIGN AND DATE THIS NOTICE.

❏ **Option 1. YES** I want to receive these items or services and get an official Medicare decision about coverage. Please submit a claim, with any evidence supporting my need for these items or services, to Medicare for its official decision. I understand you will notify me when my claim is submitted and that you will not bill me for these items or services until Medicare makes its decision. If Medicare denies payment, I agree to be personally and fully responsible for payment. That is, I will pay personally, either out of pocket or through any other insurance that I have.

I understand that I can appeal if Medicare decides not to pay. Medicare will send me notice of its official decision not to pay that explains its decision in my case. That notice will explain how I can appeal Medicare's decision not to pay. If I do not hear from Medicare about its official coverage decision within 90 days, I can telephone Medicare at: (_____)_____. TTY/TDD: (_____)_____.

❏ **Option 2. YES** I want to receive these items or services. Do NOT submit a claim to Medicare. I agree to be fully and personally responsible for payment of any amount for which my other insurance will not pay. I realize I cannot appeal to Medicare.

❏ **Option 3. NO** I will not receive these items or services. I understand that you will not be able to submit a claim to Medicare and that I will not be able to appeal your opinion that Medicare won't pay.

Patient's Name	Medicare # (HICN)
Signature of the patient or of the authorized representative	Date

Form CMS-20014 (XX/2004)   OMB Exempt

Internal Communication

Internal communication among staff members is just as important as communicating with residents and families. Some forms of internal communications may include a billing log and/or a triple check process.

Monthly billing verification/triple check

Often, if a SNF is using an electronic medical record (EMR), the formal triple check may not be necessary depending on the built-in checks and balances of the EMR. However, some form of monthly compliance log should be developed and established even with the use of an EMR. Parameters should be established surrounding who is responsible for completing each section of the log, as the responsibility should not rest with only one individual. Most models require both the RNAC and medical records staff to complete the log and submitting to the billing department for review and comparison prior to claim submission.

The following items should be part of the monthly billing verification process, at a minimum, prior to claim submission and can be formulated into a log for ease of communication between departments:

- Three-digit RUG taken from the validation report received upon acceptance of the MDS into the state database

- Assessment modifier for billing purposes (see Chapter 4, Figure 4.2)

- ARD

- Date MDS transmission was accepted by the state database

- Date span covered by the RUG and number of billable days

- Verification of the following signatures and/or completed forms:

  - Physician orders

  - Physician certification and recertification

  - Therapy plans of treatment

- Review of the following documentation to support skilled services:

  - Nurses notes

  - Therapy notes

- Therapy ARD, days, and minutes reviewed

- Diagnosis from the MDS

- Confirmation that the MDS has been signed

In addition to identifying who is responsible for verification of each item, a timeline to hold all members of the team accountable is also necessary. Similar to the month-end close process for financial purposes, the nursing and medical records department should also have a month-end close process, and verification of all of the items identified previously need to be part of that process. The triple check should really occur throughout the month, not just when it is time to bill. That said, requiring verification of the previously referenced items by the third working day of the month should not be an issue. However, often facilities require such information to be completed and submitted to the billing department by the fifth working day because the ancillary charges from outside vendors are often not provided until that date.

Should Other Residents Be Discussed?

Many times we lose sight of other residents that need to be reviewed monthly and/or periodically who may not be using the Medicare Part A benefit in the SNF.

HMO and managed care

It is a good idea to mirror the review process used for Medicare Part A residents for HMO and managed care residents as well. These residents can also be discussed during the weekly meetings and their records reviewed as part of the nursing and medical records month-end close process.

Benefits exhaust

A benefits exhaust situation occurs when a resident continues to meet the criteria for skilled services under Medicare Part A, but has exhausted the current 100-day benefit period, and Medicare Part A is no longer paying for the care in the SNF. There are special requirements SNF staff must follow to communicate the continuation of skilled services to Medicare Part A for purposes of tracking the benefit period and the 60-day break in skilled services. For these reasons, it is good practice to continue to discuss these residents' skilled services during the weekly meetings and on the monthly billing verification log to ensure that the billing department knows whether the resident is continuing skilled services or has dropped to a nonskilled level of care, both of which are required to be communicated to Medicare on a monthly basis.

Medicare Part B

It is important to perform a modified triple check for Medicare Part B residents prior to submission of the claim as well. Although Medicare Part B is not an inpatient benefit and is based on individual services billed (e.g., therapy), ensuring that all signatures, documentation, and diagnosis codes are present and consistent is crucial prior to billing.

Although less formal communication should occur on a daily basis between the IDT, the areas identified are a great starting point for a SNF who is unsure of what communication is required as well as what communication is "best practice."

CHAPTER
6

Other Important Things to Know

As this book comes to a close, there are a few more important items that do not necessarily fit into the skilled services discussion, but warrant some general discussion related to skilled nursing facility (SNF) operations. This final chapter will discuss the following:

- Medicare myths

- Consolidated billing

- Responding to medical review

Medicare Myths

Myth #1: A psychiatric resident will not qualify for Medicare Part A skilled services.
Although most psychiatric services will not qualify as Medicare Part A skilled services, there are some instances when a resident will qualify coming straight from the hospital, at least for a short period of time.

As we discussed in Chapter 2, first you need to determine if the stay in the psychiatric hospital meets the three-day qualifying hospital requirement. If it does, the next area to review is whether the care meets the requirements for skilled services under Medicare Part A.

The resident may need to have his or her medications adjusted; there also can be potential for an adverse drug reaction if medications were changed. In addition, depending on the time spent in the hospital, there may have been some deterioration and the resident may have therapy orders upon discharge from the hospital. Other areas to review include hearing, speech and vision (Section B of the minimum data set [MDS]); cognitive patterns (Section C); mood (Section D); behavior (Section E); functional status (Section G); and medications (Section N) … just to name a few!

Myth #2: You can cover a resident for the first five days to observe and assess his or her condition.

The Centers for Medicare & Medicaid Services (CMS) provides no time frame of minimum or maximum time covered; however, as discussed in Chapter 3 of this book, there is the ability to use administrative presumption of coverage. Remember, though, that the use of the administrative presumption is reserved only for residents being directly admitted from a three-day qualifying hospital stay. In addition, this administrative presumption only covers up to and including the assessment reference date (ARD) if no skilled need is identified on the initial admission/readmission MDS. The regulation, as discussed in Chapter 3, indicates that a resident can be skilled "until the condition of the patient is stabilized." Typically, skilled care for observation and assessment lasts for a few weeks or less.

Myth #3: A new diagnosis triggers a new benefit period.

This is one of the most dangerous Medicare myths out there! It can impact not only resident care, but also customer service and can have a significant financial impact as well. The only way a resident can earn a new 100-day benefit period under SNF Medicare Part A is to complete a 60-day period of wellness, as discussed in Chapter 2. The calculation for earning a new benefit period is based on two criteria:

1. Determining when skilled services ended

2. Counting days

There is no magic formula to earning a new benefit period. Let us review an example to illustrate how the calculation should work.

> Resident completed a 100-day Medicare benefit period on December 31. Resident remained skilled under Medicare Part B, receiving therapy services until January 31. Beginning February 1, the resident was no longer at a skilled level of care. Based on the counting of 60 days, the resident would be eligible for a new benefit period on April 2 (assuming 28 days in February). However, we need to review each day between February 1 and April 2 to make sure none of the following occurred:
>
> *   *Did the resident receive any services that would qualify the resident under a Medicare skilled level of care while in the SNF during that time period? For example, was the resident picked back up under a Medicare Part B plan of care that met the skilled level of care requirements?*
>
> *   *Did the resident have any inpatient admissions to the hospital during that time period?*

If the answer to either of these questions is yes, then the resident did not earn a new 100-day benefit period based on either the provision of skilled services or failure to meet the 60-day period of wellness requirement.

There is one small wrinkle in this calculation of benefit periods. If a resident leaves the SNF and continues to receive a skilled service while residing at home, for example, this would not impact the benefit period. When reviewing skilled services received, Medicare is only looking at skilled services received while in a SNF or as an inpatient of a hospital. Skilled services rendered to a beneficiary in the home setting do not impact the Medicare Part A SNF benefit period calculation.

Myth #4: All residents who are receiving tube feeding are always skilled and always will be skilled. This statement is both true and false. The caveat lies with the level of calories and fluid the resident is taking in through the tube. As we discussed in Chapter 4, residents who meet the 26%–50% of calories and 501cc of fluid per day via the feeding tube, or residents who receive 51% or more of calories via the feeding tube will automatically qualify for Medicare Part A benefits in a SNF. Additionally, they are required to continue on Medicare to use a full 100-day benefit period until they drop below such levels on an MDS. These levels will also continue that spell of illness and prevent the resident from attaining the 60-day period of wellness to qualify for a new 100-day benefit period.

Residents who meet the caloric and fluid requirements of 26%–50% of caloric intake and 501cc of fluid daily via the tube or residents who receive 51% of more of caloric intake from the tube will remain at a skilled level of care for a full 100 days, as long as they remain at those levels. In addition, the resident will not qualify for a new 100-day benefit period unless he or she:

- Drops below the calorie and fluid levels previously identified for 60 consecutive days without any other skilled service in the SNF or inpatient hospital stay

- Remains at those calorie and fluid levels identified previously but discharges to home with skilled services being provided in the home for 60 consecutive days

Myth #5: As long as there is an inpatient hospital stay or Medicare Part A SNF stay within the last 30 days, we can pick the resident back up on Medicare Part A.
Although this is partly true, the most important criteria to using the 30-day window as discussed in Chapter 2 is relating the reason for coverage back to the original hospitalization or a condition that

arose during treatment. If the reason to pick the resident back up under Medicare Part A is completely unrelated to the original hospitalization or subsequent SNF stay, the criteria outlined in the regulation regarding the 30-day transfer rules are not met, and the resident should not be put back on Medicare Part A.

Myth #6: A resident on Medicare Part A in a SNF can never leave the SNF for an overnight leave of absence.

As discussed in Chapter 3, often, a resident is unable to leave the SNF due to the complexity of the services being rendered in the SNF. That said, a couple of items need to be reviewed before determining if an overnight leave of absence (LOA) is feasible.

1. Can the resident safely be away from the SNF and can the family or responsible party be taught to safely meet the resident's needs while out of the SNF?

2. Are the absences infrequent in nature and not for prolonged periods of time?

Obviously, question one is important to make sure that the resident can be properly cared for during the LOA. It is always necessary to consult with the resident's physician to notify him or her of the LOA request and get some feedback from the physician's point of view on whether the LOA is feasible. The second question relates more to being sure that the practical matter criteria also discussed in Chapter 3 is being met. If a resident is able to leave the SNF on a weekly basis for an overnight visit, or if the resident leaves for prolonged periods of time three times per week to attend an off-site bingo game, for example, it is doubtful that the practical matter criteria is being met. Remember, one of the four criteria related to meeting the skilled services requirement in a SNF is the practical matter criteria identified in Section 30.7 of the *Medicare Benefit Policy Manual* (Pub. 100-02):

- *As a practical matter, considering economy and efficiency, the daily skilled services can be provided only on an inpatient basis in a SNF (see §30.7).*

That said, although a resident may safely be able to go on LOAs frequently or for prolonged periods of time, the question becomes: Is the SNF the most appropriate place for that resident to receive those skilled services?

Consolidated Billing

Looking back, it is hard to believe that the concept of SNF consolidated billing (CB) has been around since 1998, yet we still struggle with some of the concepts. That being said, let us quickly review the basics before we get into some of the areas with which SNF staff seem to struggle.

Back to basics

In 1997, the Balanced Budget Act (BBA) was written into law, as discussed in Chapter 1 of this book. A large component of the BBA for SNFs was the introduction to CB. The BBA mandated that most services provided to SNF residents in a Medicare Part A stay be included in the Part A resource utilization group (RUG) rate. This mandate precluded outside vendors from billing services separately to Medicare Part B for residents in a SNF Medicare Part A stay. This mandate served the following three main purposes:

- To reduce the amount of money beneficiaries were paying for services (residents were paying not only the coinsurance on their Part A SNF stay, but also on the Part B services being billed by the outside vendors during the same time period)

- To eliminate the potential for duplicate billing of services by multiple providers

- To require the SNF to take a more active role in the coordination of care for its Medicare Part A residents

As of the publication of this book, CB can either apply to a specific provider type or a specific category of service as identified by CMS.

What about Medicare Part B—Does Consolidated Billing Apply?

Consolidated billing does apply to Medicare Part B in a SNF. However, the only items that are consolidated are therapy services: physical and occupational therapy and speech-language pathology services. Any other services provided by an outside vendor including, but not limited to, laboratory, radiology, and ambulance transportation for a non-Medicare Part A resident are billed directly to Medicare by the vendor. However, therapy services, whether provided by the SNF or a hospital, are required to be billed by the SNF.

Current provider exclusions include the following:

- Physicians

- Physician assistants

- Nurse practitioners

- Clinical nurse specialists

- Certified nurse mid-wives

- Qualified psychologists

- Certified RN anesthetists

- Hospice care related to a terminal illness

- Ambulance providers (only for certain services, as discussed later in this section)

Ambulance transportation requires further explanation. Before you can determine if the services are excluded, the services must first be medically reasonable and necessary. The best way to determine this is to look at the following criteria:

1. Resident is bed-confined

2. Resident is non–weight-bearing

3. Resident cannot safely travel via any other means of transportation

Once the ambulance transportation is deemed medically reasonable and necessary, there are only three situations when the SNF would be responsible for paying for ambulance transportation.

1. A trip home if the resident returns by midnight

2. A trip from one SNF to another for admission purposes (SNF A pays for the transportation to SNF B)

3. A round trip to or from a diagnostic or therapeutic site other than an outpatient hospital setting or dialysis facility (e.g., physician office, radiation clinic, chemotherapy clinic)

A good rule of thumb to apply in all cases, except in major category III, is that if the service is excluded, the ambulance transportation is also excluded. A good example is radiation therapy. When provided at a hospital, the radiation therapy is excluded, as is the ambulance transportation. When provided at a clinic, the radiation therapy is not excluded, nor is the ambulance transportation.

Major Categories of Items and Services

CMS has further broken down specific items and services into five major categories to assist providers in understanding what is included and what is excluded from SNF CB.

Major category I

The items and services listed in this category have to be provided on an outpatient basis at a hospital in order to be excluded. CMS feels that the hospital is the most equipped venue to handle providing these services to Medicare beneficiaries. If provided at any other location, such as a clinic or physician office, the service is not excluded and the SNF is responsible for payment.

- CT scans

- Cardiac catheterizations

- MRIs

- Radiation therapy

- Angiography

- Outpatient surgery

- Emergency room services

Major category II

These items and services have to be provided by specific providers and only to specific beneficiaries as follows: must be provided to end-stage renal disease (ESRD) beneficiaries or beneficiaries who have elected the hospice benefit; and must be provided by a dialysis or hospice provider.

- Dialysis supplies

- Dialysis equipment

- Erythropoietin (EPO)

- Hospice care for terminally ill residents

Major category III

These items and services are only required to be provided by Medicare providers licensed to provide them. However, the tricky part comes in when you consider that these items and services are not categorical exclusions. What that means is that not all services that fall under these service categories are excluded. Each item or service provided will have to be looked up individually to be sure of the exclusion or inclusion status. (Resources for this are discussed later in this section.)

- Chemotherapy

- Chemotherapy administration

- Radioisotopes

- Customized prosthetic devices

Major category IV

Although these services are excluded from Medicare Part A, they can only be billed to Medicare Part B by the SNF. The outside vendor providing the service has to bill the SNF, and the SNF submits a claim to Medicare for reimbursement of these services outside of the RUG rate.

- Mammograms

- Vaccines and vaccine administration

- Pap smears and pelvic examinations

- Colorectal screenings

- Prostate screenings

- Glaucoma screenings

Medicare looks at items in category IV as preventative and diagnostic in nature. Services that fall into that category are considered Part B reimbursable items, which is why they are required to be billed to Medicare Part B outside of the RUG rate.

Major category V

This category refers to the services covered under Medicare Part B consolidated billing and includes all physical and occupational therapy services, as well as speech-language pathology services, regardless of where the services were provided to the resident (SNF or hospital).

FIGURE 6.1   **Road map to SNF consolidated billing information**

Road map to SNF Consolidated Billing Information using the CMS website at *www.cms.hhs.gov*

Medicare

Billing: SNF Consolidated Billing

Overview

Resources

CMS has put together an extensive list of resources and materials on their website.

From this site, you can access resources that will provide you with guidance on the following:

- An overview of the SNF CB program and some additional background information

- Fiscal intermediary (FI)/A/B MAC update files back several years

- Carrier A/B MAC update files back several years

Responding to Medical Reviews

In order to successfully respond to a medical review request, you need to have a process for every aspect of the response. Identify and assign specific action steps for each department involved. Without a streamlined process in place with accountability for all staff members involved, the negative impact to your bottom line could be significant.

Timelines for return of requested records

In most cases, timelines can vary from either 30 days from the date of the request or 45 days from the date of the request. However, with some Medicare Advantage (MA) medical reviews, the timeline can be as little as 14 days from the date of the request.

Notification

Based on the growing number of entities requesting records and types of reviews, it is important to understand that notification/request for records can come in different forms. For most progressive correction action (PCA) claims, the notification comes in the form of a specific claim status on the Fiscal Intermediary Shared System (FISS) a few days after a claim is successfully transmitted to Medicare. This claim status will be SB6000 or SB6001. However, for most other traditional Medicare and MA review types, a formal letter is sent to the SNF via regular mail. What is difficult about this method is that it can be addressed to a specific person, a specific job title, or a specific department.

Putting a Process Together

Identify the team

At a minimum, the medical review team should include billing, nursing, MDS, medical records, and administration. For example, the team may include the biller, director of nursing, MDS coordinator, health information manager, and administrator. A team including these players will ensure that all bases are covered related to notification, document collection, document review, and final submission of the request.

Develop an accountability checklist

The date of the notice should be counted as day one of the process with the request being mailed, allowing enough time to be logged in by the reviewing entity prior to the due date of the request. Please see Figure 6.2 for an example checklist for a 45-day record request. This will ensure that all parties are aware of the timetable and will note who is accountable for each step in the process.

Develop a record checklist. Depending on whether the request is for an inpatient or outpatient claim, the checklist will differ. Please see figures 6.3 and 6.4 for an example of a SNF Medicare Part A record request checklist and a Medicare Part B record request checklist, respectively.

However, it is important to make sure that documentation only relevant to the dates of service being billed on the claim are included. Another step in the process is to make sure someone other than the staff member who compiled the response packet reviews the information. The second page of each documentation checklist provides some guidance regarding what the reviewer should be looking for in the documentation.

FIGURE 6.2   Example checklist for 45-day record request

Medical Review Timeline and Template—45-day Request

Campus: Date of Request   1/1/11

Month of Claims:

Step / Action Step	Timeline	Staff Accountable	Specific Campus Dates
Notification of review to national director of healthcare (NDH) from central office billing staff. NDH will provide a timeline to campus staff. a. Central office billing staff member will provide notification of date put into review status including roster of claims including resident name, Medicare number, and dates of service.	Day 1	Central office billing staff	1/1/11
Campus staff to review and print required documentation and draft cover letters for all residents using the template per CRC Policy 2800.	Day 1–15	Campus clinical and therapy staff	1/15/11
All resident materials to be copied and sent overnight express mail to outside consultant for review.	Day 15	Director of nursing/ HIM	1/15/11
Campus staff to review materials for documentation consistency and completeness.	Day 16–25	Campus clinical and therapy staff	1/25/11
Outside consultant to review materials for documentation consistency and completeness.	Day 16–25	Outside consultant	1/25/11
Outside consultant report due back to campus via e-mail and conference call schedule to review.	Day 25	Outside consultant/ campus clinical and therapy staff/CRC H&W representative	
Campus staff to review outside consultant memo, complete resident information packets, revise cover letter(s), and prepare for mailing to entity requesting information.	Day 25–35	Campus clinical and therapy staff	2/4/11
Campus to mail all materials to entity requesting information.	Day 35	Healthcare administrator/DON	2/4/11
Prepay probe materials must be at the requesting entity office by the 44th day at the very latest.*	Day 44		2/13/11

*Check to ensure this calculated date does not fall on a weekend; if it does, adjust due date

Please attach roster of claims

FIGURE
6.3

Part A documentation checklist

Medical Review Documentation Checklist
Part A/Inpatient Claim

Resident name: _____   Time period in review: _____

ADR document received: _____   ADR documents due: _____

Part I: Initial documentation collection

Documents			
Requested	**N/A**	**Date gathered**	**Detailed List**
			Notes with supporting documentation for 30 days prior to the ARD
			Hospital discharge summaries
			Transfer forms
			Physician orders
			Physician admission H&P
			Physician progress notes
			Physician certification and recertifications
			Patient care plans
			MDS for each time period identified on the covered claim
			Nursing notes
			Nursing rehabilitation notes
			Therapy evaluation for each discipline provided
			Therapy reevaluation for each discipline provided, if applicable
			Plans of treatment for each discipline provided
			Therapy progress notes
			Therapy service treatment grids for each discipline provided
			Nursing rehabilitation records
			Medication records
			Treatment records
			Flow charts
			Vital sign records
			Weight charts
			Lab and other test results

FIGURE 6.3 Part A documentation checklist (cont.)

Requested	N/A	Date gathered	Detailed List
			Other documentation supporting need for the skilled services being provided in the SNF (i.e., resident services meetings)
			Only send information that is relevant to the dates being reviewed or to support MDS ARD.
Date:			Signed:
Date:			Signed:

Medical Review Documentation Checklist
Part A/Inpatient Claim

Resident name: _____ Time period in review: _____

ADR document received: _____ ADR documents due: _____

Place a check mark (✓) next to the documents requested.

Part II: Review of Documentation Collected

Documents			
Requested	N/A	Date gathered	Detailed List
			To be reviewed by two parties before packet is sent:
			Copy of the request letter and what is in the packet being compiled
			No service was started until a physician order was obtained
			All ordered services were administered; if not, there is a note to indicate why
			MDS schedule was transmitted to the state repository
			MDS schedule was followed
			Level of care requirement was met
			Services were "reasonable and necessary"
			Documentation of the medical necessity for Medicare coverage supports the coding on the MDS and the need for services rendered
			Nursing documentation indicates improvement in functional abilities
			Therapy notes indicate progress
			Therapy and nursing notes are congruent for patient participation and acceptance
			Does the MDS support the need for therapy interventions?
			Do the therapy logs with the number of days and minutes match the MDS coding?
Date:			Signed:
Date:			Signed:

FIGURE 6.4	Part B documentation checklist

Medical Review Documentation Checklist
Part B/Outpatient Claim

Resident name: _____   Time period in review: _____

ADR document received: _____   ADR documents due: _____

Part I: Initial documentation collection

Documents			
Requested	**N/A**	**Date gathered**	**Detailed List**
			Physician orders for each discipline provided
			Therapy service treatment grids for each discipline provided
			Initial evaluations and re-evaluations for each discipline provided
			Plans of treatment for each discipline provided
			Physician progress notes
			Therapy progress notes
			Nurses notes
			Lab and other test results
			Other documentation supporting need for the skilled services being provided in the SNF (i.e., resident services meetings)
			Only send information that is relevant to the dates being reviewed
Date:		**Signed:**	
Date:		**Signed:**	

FIGURE
6.4

Part B documentation checklist (cont.)

Medical Review Documentation Checklist
Part B/Outpatient Claim

Resident name: _____ Time period in review: _____

ADR document received: _____ ADR documents due: _____

Place a check mark (✓) next to the documents requested.

Part II: Review of Documentation Collected

Documents			
Requested	**N/A**	**Date gathered**	**Detailed List**
			To be reviewed by two parties before packet is sent:
			Does the documentation indicate when a decline was noted?
			Does the documentation indicate any cause of the decline?
			Does the documentation indicate whether nontherapy interventions were initiated?
			Does the documentation indicate decline and justification for skilled treatment?
			Does the documentation indicate that the physician was called and ordered an evaluation?
			When order obtained, does it indicate decline and justification for skilled treatment?
			Ensure therapy has signed plan of treatment.
			Does the documentation indicate when a decline was noted?
			Does the documentation indicate any cause of the decline?
			Does the documentation indicate whether nontherapy interventions were initiated?
			Does the documentation indicate decline and justification for skilled treatment?
			Does the documentation indicate that the physician was called and ordered an evaluation?
			When order obtained, does it indicate decline and justification for skilled treatment?
Date:			**Signed:**
Date:			**Signed:**

Avoid common pitfalls

One area that most SNF staff struggle with is the timing of the record submission. For example, if the requesting party is the fiscal intermediary (FI) and the records are due 11/1/10, the records should be mailed at least seven days in advance. With the FI, the records may be requested to be sent to a post office box, where they are opened and logged. Staff must allow time for that logging process to happen; mailing the documents in this instance on 10/31/10 will cause the claims to reject for failure to submit documents in a timely manner. When records are not able to be sent via an overnight service, I would recommend sending the documents one week before the due date and use a tracking system to mail the documents, such as certified mail or return-receipt requested.

Another area that causes trouble in a SNF is not properly identifying the team members or not holding team members accountable. One person should be designated as the manager of the process. This is not necessarily the person with the most accountability within the various tasks, and really, it should not be that person. Having a billing staff member designated as the manager is a good choice in most cases, as he or she will start the process when the claim is flagged for medical review or a letter is received from the requesting party. In addition, he or she will not be gathering or reviewing records, but can keep the accountability checklist alive and follow up with the other team members to keep the process on track.

FREE HEALTHCARE COMPLIANCE AND MANAGEMENT RESOURCES!

Need to control expenses yet stay current with critical issues?

Get timely help with FREE e-mail newsletters from HCPro, Inc., the leader in healthcare compliance education. Offering numerous free electronic publications covering a wide variety of essential topics, you'll find just the right e-newsletter to help you stay current, informed, and effective. All you have to do is sign up!

With your FREE subscriptions, you'll also receive the following:

- Timely information, to be read when convenient with your schedule
- Expert analysis you can count on
- Focused and relevant commentary
- Tips to make your daily tasks easier

And here's the best part: There's no further obligation—just a complimentary resource to help you get through your daily challenges.

It's easy. Visit *www.hcmarketplace.com/free/e-newsletters* to register for as many free e-newsletters as you'd like, and let us do the rest.

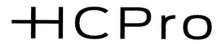

HCPro | Insight for healthcare compliance and management